Writing for Health Care Professions

Other books of interest

The Royal Marsden Hospital
Manual of Clinical Nursing Procedures
A. Phylip Pritchard and Jane Mallett
0 632 03387 8

The Royal Marsden Hospital
Manual of Standards of Care
Joanna M. Luthert and Lorraine Robinson
0 632 03386 X

The Research Process in Nursing
Second Edition
Desmond F.S. Cormack
0 632 02891 2

Health Care Research by Degrees
Norma Reid
0 632 03466 1

MRI in Practice
Catherine Westbrook and Carolyn Kaut
0 632 03587 0

Neuropsychology for Occupational Therapists
June Grieve
0 632 03303 7

Collaborative Care
Sally Hornby
0 632 03725 3

Sociology of Health and Health Care
Steve Taylor and David Field
0 632 03402 5

Health Promotion
Alison Dines and Alan Cribb
0 632 03543 9

Writing For Health Care Professions

DESMOND F.S. CORMACK
PhD, MPhil, DipEd, DipNurs, RMN, RGN
Honorary Reader in Health and Nursing
Department of Health and Nursing
Queen Margaret College
Clerwood Terrace
Edinburgh EH12 8TS

WITH CONTRIBUTIONS FROM

DAVID C. BENTON
BSc, MPhil, RGN, RMN
Director of Quality and Community Relations
East London & The City Health Authority

OXFORD

BLACKWELL SCIENTIFIC PUBLICATIONS

LONDON EDINBURGH BOSTON

MELBOURNE PARIS BERLIN VIENNA

© 1994 by
Blackwell Scientific Publications
Editorial Offices:
Osney Mead, Oxford OX2 0EL
25 John Street, London WC1N 2BL
23 Ainslie Place, Edinburgh, EH3 6AJ
238 Main Street, Cambridge,
    Massachusetts 02142, USA
54 University Street, Carlton,
    Victoria 3053, Australia

Other Editorial Offices:
Librairie Arnette SA
1, rue de Lille
75007 Paris
France

Blackwell Wissenschafts-Verlag GmbH
Düsseldorfer Str. 38
D-10707 Berlin
Germany

Blackwell MZV
Feldgasse 13
A-1238 Wien
Austria

First published under the title
    *Writing for Nursing and Allied
    Professions* 1984
Second edition entitled *Writing for Health
    Care Professions* published 1994

Set by DP Photosetting, Aylesbury, Bucks
Printed and bound in Great Britain by
Biddles Ltd, Guildford, Surrey

DISTRIBUTORS

Marston Book Services Ltd
PO Box 87
Oxford OX2 0DT
(*Orders*: Tel: 0865 791155
          Fax: 0865 791927
          Telex: 837515)

USA
Blackwell Scientific Publications, Inc.
238 Main Street
Cambridge, MA 02142
(*Orders*: Tel: 800 759-6102
               617 876-7000)

Canada
Times Mirror Professional Publishing, Ltd
130 Flaska Drive
Markham, Ontario L6G 1B8
(*Orders*: Tel: 800 268-4178
               416 470-6739)

Australia
Blackwell Scientific Publications Pty Ltd
54 University Street,
Carlton, Victoria 3053
(*Orders*: Tel: 03 347-5552)

British Library
Cataloguing in Publication Data

A catalogue record for this book is available
from the British Library

ISBN 0-632-03449-1

Library of Congress
Cataloging in Publication Data
Cormack, Desmond.
    Writing for health care professions /
Desmond F.S. Cormack, with contributions
from David C. Benton.—2nd ed.
        p.   cm.
    Rev. ed. of: Writing for nursing and allied
professions. 1984.
    Includes bibliographical references and
index.
    ISBN 0–632–03449–1
    1. Medical writing.   2. Nursing—
Authorship.   I. Benton, David C.
II. Cormack, Desmond.   Writing for
nursing and allied professions.
III. Title.
    [DNLM: 1. Writing.   WZ 345 C811w
1994]
R119.C64   1994
808'.06661—dc20   93–31924
                                   CIP

Contents

Prologue

An important feature of any profession is the extent to which its members contribute to the development of its literature. Indeed, such a contribution is a key feature of professionalism. In addition to developing skills in this area of writing, some individuals also wish to develop others including the ability to write talks, research proposals and reports, curriculum vitae, book reviews and so on. This text has been prepared for professionals who wish to develop a variety of writing skills, including those required for publication. It is not intended to be a blueprint for style or structure: rather it is a set of general guidelines. Readers will be aware of the need to obtain and comply with the specific requirements, guidelines and specifications of the individual, organization or publishing house for whom written work is being prepared.

This book has been created to meet the needs of all health care professional groups in the firm belief that the same general principles apply irrespective of discipline. It is for use by physiotherapists, dentists, doctors, occupational therapists, nurses, chiropodists, midwives, clinical psychologists, pharmacists, social workers and all other health care groups who increasingly use and contribute to each others' literature. It is intended to have equal application to clinicians, managers, researchers and teachers.

Apart from the 'Recommended Reference Texts' at the end of the book, no references to previously published works are included. The references which have been used in the text have been invented for illustration only.

Because of the uniqueness of each writer's style, it would be wrong to regard this book as a model of writing style; the style used in this book is unique to those who wrote it. Rather, the purpose is to discuss techniques that will ensure the best presentation, structure and readability. In short, it will help readers develop their personal style.

Another purpose of the book is to present and discuss the many publishing opportunities that are available to members of the professions, and how to utilize these. *All* health care professionals are capable of the many forms of writing presented here, including writing for publication, are motivated to do so, and have something important to write about. The block for many is a lack of information about the mechanics of writing and of how to get excellent ideas on paper and subsequently published.

None of the chapters can be fully utilized without some reference to a number of others. For example, in relation to 'Articles' (Chapter 15), 'Research Reports' (Chapter 13) and 'Dissertations and Theses' (Chapter 14), useful material will also be found in 'Writing Style and Structure' (Chapter 4), 'Illustrations' (Chapter 8) and 'Literature Review' (Chapter 7).

Chapter 1
Writing and Professionalism

All health care professionals, and those in training, use writing skills at some point in their career. For some, apart from writing brief clinical reports for example, developing this skill begins and virtually ends during basic training. For others it is a lifetime commitment. Some develop writing ability in a personalized and self-taught way; others receive formal preparation. Most students in the health care professions produce large amounts of coursework in essay form, and are given a variable quality of educational assistance for this. Some do well without such help; many struggle. Perhaps it is assumed that writing skills are possessed by all people who have recently left school and have entered the professions. This assumption is wrong on two counts. First, many school leavers do not have the level of writing skill required by the professions. Secondly, some students left school many years earlier and are more than a little rusty.

Exams and coursework apart, all health professionals have an obligation to contribute to the professional literature throughout their career. Unless this is taken seriously, the literature will be dominated by the minority who are either natural writers or who have worked at developing the skill. It is also appropriate that the professions, which are numerically dominated by clinicians and practitioners, should contribute fully to the literature along with academics, researchers and managers, for each has a specialist contribution to make. Writing is not the elitist activity it once was: all disciplines and grades of staff are increasingly able to make a contribution.

This text is based on the premise that *all* health care professionals feel a duty to contribute to the literature upon which the development of their profession is based. This assumes that published literature is the heart of a profession, and that without it the profession does not exist. The ability to write for publication can be formally developed during basic professional education using essays and other forms of course-work as the basis of that development. Although teaching staff on professional courses are in an ideal position to develop writing skills in students, not all of them have the necessary experience.Where this is so, remedial action will ensure that a suitable level of skill is achieved by all health care teaching staff and through them by their students.

Beginners might assume that editors will not be interested in their manuscripts, perhaps because they do not have a string of academic or professional qualifications. This view is mistaken: most health professionals do not have numerous qualifications, particularly at the early stage of a career.

Some individuals feel that they do not have time to write, being too involved in *doing* the job to find time to write about it. Such a view might be acceptable in the short term in that it enables concentration on clinical work for example. However, in the longer term this view is at odds with professionalism in that it prevents dissemination of valued knowledge.

Although writing undoubtedly offers personal rewards such as the sense of achievement from having something published, career enhancement, and occasional modest financial rewards, the major rewards are much greater than the personal ones. These come from having contributed to the development of the profession.

Thus, there is a duty for all professionals in all disciplines, irrespective of level of experience or number of postbasic qualifications, to become involved in some aspect of writing for publication. Although this view is intentionally uncompromising, it is appreciated that developing the necessary skills poses difficulties for some individuals. The purpose of this book is to minimize these difficulties and help make the best use of personal writing potential.

WHY PUBLISH?

All qualified staff will have experience of coursework and writing for examinations. The importance of this type of writing is not to be underestimated as everyone will have achieved a measure of success with or without formal help available as part of the professional course. Some will be involved in writing as part of a work commitment, for personal project work, or for employer-commissioned projects, for example. Others will continue to write for educational purposes in postbasic courses including research-based dissertations.

Perhaps the greatest opportunity for writing is in contributing to the professional literature. This is done for a number of reasons, as follows.

- *To inform:* There is a clear need for professionals to inform others about how they understand their profession in terms of clinical practice, research, education and management. The 'how it is done' paper may be based on personal experience or opinion, or may have a research base. All health professionals profit from examining their activity closely and asking themselves 'Do I do or know something which may be of value to others?'.
- *To educate:* Professional education comes from two distinct sources: from the college or university, and from clinical/practical

experience. To a greater or lesser degree, theoretical classroom-based material does not quite match the reality of what occurs in the workplace. Part of this dichotomy results from some textbooks being written by those who have relatively little recent and direct clinical contact. It is therefore essential that clinicians in all disciplines play a significant part in contributing to the literature used by the health professions.

- *To speculate and predict:* The health care professions, which are relatively conservative, probably need to do more to encourage those individuals who see the future and development of their profession in a way which is 'different' from the majority view. Such people are sometimes branded as radicals or deviants. Although the encouragement of speculation and prediction results in a degree of uncertainty, tolerance of those willing and able to make this unique and most valuable contribution to health care is desirable. Professionals who march to a different tune can do much to secure the future of their profession.

- *To question and challenge:* The ability of individuals to question and challenge subjects and decisions relating to their profession is a healthy sign. All professionals have the right, indeed obligation, to seriously challenge individuals or groups who make public pronouncements about their profession. This type of writing frequently takes the form of published interviews and letters to, or news items in, professional journals.

- *To raise issues:* One way of highlighting important professional issues and to draw them to the attention of others is to write for publication. All professionals have the right, the experience and the duty to raise issues for public debate. In the past the discussion of major issues, and the proposed solutions, have often been left to committees, academics and managers. These individuals and groups, although an important part of the professions, would not claim to have a monopoly in the discussion of relevant issues or proposed solutions.

  Once major issues are raised by individuals, others can then contribute to the public debate. Clearly, the development of an appropriate level of writing skill will enable the presentation of a much stronger and more reasoned contribution.

- *To influence opinion:* Although the opinion of individuals and groups is often shaped by personal experience, other factors play a part. The written word is a powerful means of influencing opinion. A well-presented and forceful argument which is either published or sent to an individual or group can play a large part in helping them understand the views of the writer. Many of the 'open letters' published by the professional press are designed deliberately to influence the opinion of all or a specific part of the readership.

- *To clarify personal ideas:* When developing a new idea in some aspect of clinical functioning, the individual might publish that idea and thereby expose it to the critical attention of a peer group. In this case the purpose of the writing is to share the idea with others and to obtain feedback from them and thus better understand, clarify and justify the ideas or proposals contained in the published material.

WHERE TO PUBLISH?

The opportunities for writing are numerous, more so than many professionals realize. Some of the major outlets for writing are discussed in this book. Others such as newspapers, non-professional journals and other non-professional publications are referred to only briefly. In the health professions the largest source of original written material is undoubtedly the hundreds of current journals. Whilst some of these relate to health care generally, there are a small number of highly specialized publications.

Health professionals additionally have much to contribute to 'lay' publications including popular magazines and newspapers. Increasingly the editors of these publications are recruiting health professionals to write regular articles, news features or other health-related items. Here, health care staff are given an opportunity to convey aspects of their work to the general public. There are also considerable opportunities for writing in the professional journals of other disciplines. Another aspect of professional literature is that it can have international applicability. Although the number is decreasing, many journals publish materials that have been written mainly by professionals residing in the country in which the journal is published. There is a need for health professionals to become more aware of the internationalization of health care and to recognize that health care staff in any part of the world have much to teach, and learn from, colleagues elsewhere. Those trying to decide how to make best use of writing skills should therefore seriously consider the international literature as a potential outlet. Provided that material is relevant to groups outside the country of its origin, a serious attempt should be made to have it exposed to as wide an international readership as possible.

The uses to which writing skills can be put are many; there is clearly a multitude of possible outlets for them. One of those that has not been mentioned here, but which is of equal importance, is the preparation and submission of written evidence to committees, groups or individuals involved in health care. The written word can also be a persuasive tool in conveying feelings to professionals and others who hold public office – Members of Parliament, for example.

WHEN TO PUBLISH

Ideally, writing should be viewed as something that should be undertaken throughout a career. It would be easy to say that the best time to write is 'when there is something to say'. However, this is not entirely true. All too often the reason given for failure to contribute to the literature is that the person cannot readily think of something about which to write. It is likely that all professionals can find, with a little effort, something in their background, knowledge or experience that deserves to be related to colleagues through the written word.

Even if a writing topic cannot be identified at present, the possibility of writing in the future should be considered. For example, when embarking on a new project or approach to clinical work, it is a good idea to record the progress of the project in such a way that it will lend itself to publication in due course. In short, the possibility of publishing in the future should always be regarded as a real one. Similarly, if a dissertation or other form of coursework is written as part of a course requirement, the writer should consider how the material might be reshaped or rewritten for publication.

Some potential writers struggle for long periods with an idea in an attempt to write about it, often unsuccessfully. This is often accompanied by a mistaken notion that perfection has to be achieved on the first attempt. Nothing can be further from the truth. With very few exceptions, written material goes into many drafts. The point here is that the would-be writer should not wait for inspiration in the hope of this producing instant perfection, but must start to write *now*. Once a start is made, it is surprising how the material can be added to, refined and shaped into a desirable end product.

PERMISSION TO PUBLISH

At the time of deciding when to write comes the need to determine whom to inform or consult or whom to ask for permission. Although there are no straightforward answers to these questions, there are some general principles which may help avoid potential pitfalls. Articles in professional journals no longer *automatically* carry a footnote in which the author thanks the head of department or senior colleague with whom he or she works, but it is still necessary to consider who should be asked, consulted or informed. Although some managers and senior colleagues may regard the writing activities of junior colleagues as being their own business, most still prefer to be informed.

As a general rule, a private and personal opinion that is expressed in writing, and contains no reference to the writer's place of work nor any information generated in and identifiable with the place of work, does not require permission to be published. If, however, the paper makes reference to a place of work, even if only in the author's biographical details, or relates to activity which is being undertaken there, then permission will usually be required. This is usually obtained from the employing authority via a line manager. Similarly, if the writer incorporates any ideas or material obtained from colleagues, these should be formally acknowledged and permission obtained from the source of the assistance. In the event of there being doubt about the need to get permission from managers or an employer, it is advisable to ask for a copy of a written policy on the subject. If it does not exist, the request may act as a prompt for its production.

It is not being suggested that employers or their agents should be given the power to give or withhold permission for professional staff to publish. However, if the publication identifies an employer or a workplace, permission may be required. If an employer or workplace is not identified, health professionals ought to be free to publish whatever they wish. This right to literary freedom is central to the concept of professionalism and must be jealously protected.

For some groups, such as those working directly for government departments, it is often a contractual requirement that the employer's permission be obtained prior to any publishing activity, whether or not the publication identifies the employer or the author's place of work, or contains information derived from working for that employer. Such a severe constraint on the publishing freedom of a professional is rather inhibiting but must be complied with. In case of doubt, it is important to ask whether or not formal permission is needed. If it is, a request must be made in writing and a written reply must be obtained as must a copy of the contractual statement which states that permission is needed.

ETHICAL AND LEGAL ISSUES

All forms of professional writing have legal or ethical aspects, often both. In considering these, particularly if the material is to be published, the writer will be guided by the publisher. However, final responsibility lies with the author. This section is not a definitive or comprehensive statement on the ethical and legal issues relating to professional publication. Rather it is intended to raise general awareness of these.

Honesty and integrity

The writer is in a privileged position in that much of what is published will be assumed by readers to be true. Although the publisher, usually through referees, checks submitted material, much has to be left to the honesty and integrity of the writer. Although that which is apparently or obviously untrue will be challenged or not be accepted, some material is difficult, if not impossible, to check. For example, it would be difficult for referees, and subsequently readers, to ascertain that research findings had been 'massaged' in order to make a research report more interesting. Similarly, information obtained from patients or colleagues in private conversations usually cannot be checked by third parties.

For better or worse, many readers assume that the written word is truthful and they are totally dependent on the honesty and integrity of the writer.

Accuracy

Readers will assume that published material is accurate and that the writer has taken all reasonable steps to ensure this. The consequences of failure to do so on the part of the writer can range from the very serious – a significant error in describing a treatment, for example – to the irritating – for example, a bibliographical error in a reference.

Whilst it is virtually impossible to ensure that there are no errors in a published item, especially in longer items such as textbooks, it is the responsibility of the author to minimize these. In particular, it is essential that no error appears which will do harm to others. The publisher may pick up errors where the text does not quite ring true, but cannot be expected to check accuracy. Errors introduced by the printer during typesetting should be detected and corrected by the publisher when the proofs are read. However, it is in the writer's own interests to ensure that they check the proofs as well as the manuscript as carefully as possible.

Libel

Libel, a false and malicious written or published statement, can result in the writer and/or publisher being sued under the laws of libel and having to apologize and pay compensation to the offended party. Libellous material may appear in a variety of formats and settings including book reviews, the 'letters page' of a journal, a limited circulation discussion document, or a book or article.

For guidance on the subject see the Society of Authors' *Quick Guide on Libel*, full details of which are in the 'Recommended reference texts' at the end of this book.

Plagiarism

Plagiarism, the appropriation of the writings or ideas of another person and passing them off as one's own, is unfortunately not unheard of in health care publishing. Whilst plagiarism is relatively easy to prove if the offender uses an identical or near identical copy of material published by someone else, it is much more difficult to detect if the plagiarized material has been suitably disguised. The professions, publishers, writers and readers rely heavily on the professional integrity of the individual to avoid plagiarism and, where the ideas or writings of others are used, to acknowledge their source.

Duplicate publication

There are rare occasions when a previously published article deserves to be published again in another journal. For example, if an article was published in a highly specialized low-circulation journal, it might subsequently be recognized that the material deserved exposure to a much wider readership via duplicate publication in a more general high-circulation journal. Providing that both journals are in agreement and readers of the second journal are informed that they are reading a duplicate publication, this arrangement is acceptable.

Duplicate publication becomes a problem when an author marginally changes a manuscript previously published in one journal and succeeds in having it published in one or more other journals without informing them that the item has been published previously. A similarly undesirable effect would be achieved by successfully submitting a number of manuscripts, all slightly different but essentially the same, to a number of journals.

In either case, undisclosed duplicate publication of identical or near identical material infringes copyright and is unethical. It may also deprive other writers of the opportunity of being able to publish because of lack of space.

Unnecessary multiple authorship

Understandably, readers usually assume that all authors of a book, chapter or article made a significant contribution to its production, whilst appreciating that some will contribute more than others. Indeed, this assumption is implicit in the criteria readers apply when evaluating a piece of work. It is therefore inappropriate for the authorship to include the names of people who made no significant contribution. Such literary parasitism, although adding to the curriculum vitae of those who agree to be included without contributing, detracts from the literary and professional credibility of all involved.

Inappropriate acknowledgement

Another form of literary parasitism is the one in which the assistance of individuals is acknowledged when in reality little or no assistance has been given. This may be done because someone, usually in a senior position, 'expects it' and might be offended if not included in the acknowledgements. Such abuse is becoming less common in that fewer people will allow an inappropriate acknowledgement of their assistance. However, abuse of position is not uncommon, and it may occasionally be necessary to yield to overt or covert pressure and act in this ethically dubious way.

Copyright infringement

Copyright is the exclusive legal right which an author or institution has to control and limit the use of their work including, but not limited to, published materials, photographs, music and so on. In particular, authors have the right to control copying of their work, and to expect those who wish to copy it to seek permission. In some cases copyright is assigned by the author to the publisher. Those wishing to reproduce such material must therefore obtain the permission of the publisher.

Copyright laws are very complex and vary from country to country. If the need to reproduce copyright material is anticipated, it would be advisable to read Clark's *Photocopying from Books and Journals* (see 'Recommended reference texts') or a similar publication.

Chapter 2
Writing Opportunities

The development of writing skills presents a unique and rewarding challenge to all health care staff at all stages of a career. Nothing in this book applies to only one or some disciplines, for the general principles apply to all groups equally.

Health professionals are no strangers to writing, since they spend a great deal of time producing clinical reports, for example. However, such material is for a relatively limited readership with whom in most instances the writer has close contact. If the reader of the clinical report should need further information or explanation, it is often possible to obtain this direct from the writer of the report. Such information is only a small part of the total information which is available. For example, if a reader is informed that 'Mr Jones is to be discharged from hospital tomorrow', they will have, or will have access to, considerable additional background knowledge of the context of that report.

In this book the phrase *writing skill* refers to a type of writing and of writing ability of which many have much less day-to-day experience. It relates to producing longer pieces of work, often but not exclusively for publication. Although many will have had the opportunity to develop writing skills during training, to fulfil coursework requirements for example, this experience is limited for two reasons. First, the skills are frequently learned by a process of trial and error. It is relatively unusual for students to be given a formal training in writing, something which is necessary to produce work of a professional and particularly of a publishable standard. Secondly, once basic professional education is complete, qualified people may fail to further develop and maintain these skills. It is not intended to imply that health professionals are unable to develop this ability: many write clinical reports daily. Rather, it is suggested that many have difficulty in writing longer pieces designed for a readership with whom they have little personal contact. This challenge is one which is faced by many professionals of all disciplines. During writing workshops that I have presented, which have been attended by staff of various grades from a number of disciplines, it has become clear that neither grade nor discipline indicates the presence or absence of writing ability. This applies equally to those with more or less professional experience.

In recent years all health professionals have become more aware of the increased expectation that they should contribute to the professional literature. The purpose of this book is to convince *all* health professionals that they have a responsibility to contribute to the literature. It is also intended to provide a number of practical guidelines, and some practical examples of how to develop the confidence and ability to write.

A few decades ago the need to write, particularly for publication, was much less apparent than it is today. The extent to which professionals in other parts of the world wished or were required to know about professional practice and events in other areas was relatively limited. However, because of the increase in the amount of professional information and knowledge in recent years, the written word is more frequently being used as a means of communicating with others. This means of communication is already well developed in some individuals in some disciplines but is by no means universally present in all professionals.

REVIEW OF WRITING OPPORTUNITIES

All professionals in all phases of their career are potential contributors to the literature. Not all literature will be for publication, some being for examination purposes, other pieces being for conference presentation, for example. Thus, professionals at all levels of experience will profit from developing their writing skills. In the case of students, such skills need not be confined to coursework and examinations. Although a beginner may be unable to add to the literature relating to clinical practice, they can say much of importance about, for example, what it is like being a student.

This review of writing opportunities, although not comprehensive, illustrates that there are a range of activities in which it is possible to become involved. They are not presented in any order of importance or in the order in which to get involved in them. For example, it is possible to become an editorial panel member without ever having written a book, book review or journal article. The writing opportunities discussed may be 'optional' in that a professional might proceed through an illustrious career without making use of them. Few individuals will become involved in all aspects of writing, even during a professional lifetime. Those who wish to write will choose the outlet which is most suited to their talent, experience and aspirations. It is often the case that a small measure of success will cause a writer to aspire to greater things, and will result in their gaining the confidence to utilize writing talents more fully.

Although some help can be given to the beginner, there is no recipe which can ensure success and there is no easy route to producing high quality written material. Some have a natural talent for producing written work, reflecting an excellent understanding of their native language; most have to work very hard to develop writing skill. However, this can be learned and all professionals should be convinced of two things: first, that success will come if one is sufficiently motivated, interested and willing to spend time in writing practice; and, secondly, that all have something unique and important to contribute to the professional literature.

Coursework and examinations

Two types of written work, coursework and examinations, are similar in that they are both submitted for exam purposes. Thus, they are both submitted to a readership with which the writer has some direct or indirect personal contact, the examiner. In general this similarity holds good although the length, depth and quality of the piece of work may vary considerably. It may range from a three-page exam answer submitted by a first-year student, to a 30-page piece of coursework submitted by a postgraduate student.

In both instances the student has made the decision to undertake the course of study for which the coursework or examination answer is required. Although this requirement may form a much larger part of one course and a relatively small part of another, they are of equal importance in that the written work must be successfully completed to achieve success in the course generally. Many students have relatively little difficulty in producing short pieces of work, for example two to three pages. However, the prospect of writing a much longer piece is a cause for concern for many. This problem is more apparent than real, and one which can be minimized by appropriate guidance and practice.

Dissertations and theses

The location of virtually all professional groups in higher education establishments has dramatically increased the frequency with which dissertations and theses are produced. These may be a requirement for diploma courses, graduate courses or higher degrees. The ability to produce longer, rather than shorter, written work is becoming an increasingly necessary feature of professional development. Many postbasic educational, clinical and managerial courses now require the extensive use of writing ability, which can thus no longer be seen as an optional extra only for those who wish to publish. All who intend to participate in the available continuing education opportunities must be able to express themselves clearly and effectively in writing.

Curriculum vitae

Soon after qualifying, perhaps earlier, every professional will want to construct a curriculum vitae (CV) or a résumé (a summary of a CV).

There are a few basic ground rules which will result in a polished and professional structure. Whereas some aspects of writing skill development are optional, writing books for example, being able to construct a CV is necessary for everyone.

Writing a speech

In the course of a career many will be given the opportunity to speak to professional audiences. For some, the opportunity is grasped immediately; for others the response is much less positive. Often the reluctance is caused by concern about writing the paper for presentation: worries about structure, length, balance and so on. This concern, if not overcome, may seriously handicap a professional career. Chapter 18 deals with this subject and offers a number of tips on the construction of a paper for presentation.

Research proposals

These will be written by a small number of people who wish to do research and therefore apply for funds, register for a higher degree, obtain permission from a research and ethics committee, or all three. Although some organizations provide an application structure by way of an application form, others do not.

Travel scholarship applications

As with research proposals, some organizations provide a structure in their application forms; others do not. In either case, there are a number of matters requiring writing skills which are rarely if ever dealt with by scholarship funding bodies: for example writing the report of the visit.

Research reports

Research by all health care professions continues to increase, making more evident the need for ability to produce well-written readable research reports. Although a minority of staff undertake and therefore write about research, the quality of the report has implications for its entire readership. A longstanding criticism of much existing research is that it is rarely read, far less implemented. Undoubtedly, the poor quality of many reports in terms of structure, presentation and readability reduces the frequency with which they are read, understood and implemented.

The prime responsibility for decisions regarding the unique content of the research report lies with the researcher and supervisors. However, the structure and presentation may be similar to those of other reports.

It is often true to say that a blueprint exists for presenting and structuring research reports, with each only requiring modifications of style.

Articles

Preparing an article for publication in a professional journal may be the first type of publishing in which to become involved. The number of articles published has escalated dramatically since the 1970s, due in a large part to the substantial growth in the number of professional journals. To survive each journal must attract an appropriate quantity and quality of articles. Many of these journals are published weekly or monthly, so the total number of professional articles published in a given year is considerable.

Some years ago the majority of articles published were written by a minority of writers who produced many articles each. This is no longer the case.

There is a myth relating to article publication which needs to be exploded. It is that most journals are so overwhelmed by submitted manuscripts that it is almost impossible for even very experienced writers to have their contributions accepted. It is surprising how many who have never submitted or prepared an article for publication labour under this illusion. The reality is that, providing a good idea is well written and well presented in the format required by the journal, getting an article published is not as difficult as many imagine. Lack of confidence is the major impediment to writing and publishing an article. In short, the average professional has the ability, and probably the motivation, to write; what is required is help in understanding the mechanics of writing and publishing.

Books

Although most professional textbooks are written by more experienced writers, there is no reason why less experienced authors should not seek the opportunity to contribute to a multiauthor text by, for example, writing a chapter on a subject which is within their area of expertise. Many books are now written by a number of authors (multiauthored books) or are compiled and edited by one person, the general editor, who seeks chapter contributions from a number of writers. Beginning writers with the appropriate level of clinical skill and experience may be contacted by a general editor who wishes to organize a book. There is no reason why a potential contributor should not contact the editor or publisher and make it known that they would be willing to write a chapter on a specific topic. Publishers are interested in hearing from potential authors who are willing either to write or to edit an entire book or to contribute to one. If a publisher is contacted by a sufficient number of individuals who, for example, feel able to contribute to a text in the same general subject area, the publisher may well put these individuals in touch with each other with a view to preparing a book on that subject.

Publishing consultancies

Some publishing companies specializing in health care journals and books have no health care professionals on their staff. Others employ one or more staff with a health background. Both groups invariably seek expert advice on specific proposals or manuscripts from professionals in one or more health-related disciplines. The advantage of this type of arrangement is that the company has access to a large and diverse range of experience and expertise. Thus, for example, if the material relates to a specialist aspect of internal medicine, a specialist in that field is consulted; if it relates to community care of the mentally ill, an expert in that field is consulted. This arrangement means that a wide range and number of health care professionals contribute to the development of professional literature.

Although many professional journals will employ full-time health professionals, they clearly cannot employ staff with every conceivable range of skill and expertise. For this reason, as with book publishers, most journals utilize the services of staff on a part-time basis, either paid or unpaid. For example a journal might have a multispeciality and/or multidisciplinary editorial panel, their function being to help in the development of the general publishing strategy and to look at submitted manuscripts.

A journal may also appoint a number of referees who will be sent submitted manuscripts for detailed examination. The referee will then recommend whether it should be accepted unchanged or, as is frequently the case, returned to the writer with suggested changes. As with publishing consultancies this involvement in the work of professional journals allows considerable numbers of clinicians, managers, educators and researchers to be actively involved in the work of professional journals.

Book reviewing

As with articles and the journals in which they appear, the number of books on or related to health care has increased manyfold in recent years. This, accompanied by the increasing cost of books, means that there is a need for a good professional reviewing system to help potential users decide which books to buy. Such a service is of vital importance to the professions, individuals, authors and publishers. It is clearly necessary to those who stock and organize professional libraries, and to those who borrow books. A book reviewing service is also of use to teachers and students, and is of considerable value to qualified staff who will maintain a small personal library throughout their career.

A book reviewing service is often one of those aspects of a professional journal which is taken for granted since readers rarely think much about the process by which books are reviewed.

Book reviewing, in common with all types of writing, requires special skills which can be learned. It is within the scope of all professionals who have developed their writing skill and who have appropriate professional experience which enables them to make informed comment.

Before discussing each of the major writing opportunities in more detail, a number of other aspects of the writing process will be discussed. The material in the next six chapters is central to the full development of writing skills.

Chapter 3
Resources for Writing

Successful writing is aided by finding, recognizing and making use of a number of resources. Beginners may feel that they must write in virtual isolation from others, for only then will the writing be unique and of real value. More experienced writers know that there are a number of resources, including people, that must be utilized for best results. Clearly, not all resources will be available to or used by an individual writer on all occasions. This chapter will show that these resources are available and should be freely used. There is certainly no need to isolate oneself from others who can be of assistance.

PROFESSIONAL EXPERIENCE

The most important resources available are training, knowledge and experience. These make the literary contribution of the professional unique. Despite their considerable importance, professional writing being impossible without them, they can be undervalued or unrecognized.

IDEAS AND INSPIRATION

Some believe that they cannot write because they have nothing to say, or because they cannot produce novel ideas. The reality is that everyone can write if they wish to do so, and that all professionals have something to write about if they wish to do so. This is not to deny that some find it easier than others. The purpose of this book is to help those who find it difficult.

A good starting point is to decide that pen *will* be put to paper, and that there is something relevant to say. The next step is to draw from professional experience and to look to it for ideas and inspiration. For example, it might seem difficult or impossible to apply a widely accepted theory to a relatively common situation, a conclusion which can only be made by a professional familiar with both the theory and its application. Now that an important idea is developing, one which challenges accepted theory, it is time to begin to write.

PREVIOUS WRITING SKILL

All professionals have developed a level of writing skill in a number of areas. Many will have written essay-type answers to exam questions; all have written essay-type answers for coursework, and clinical reports on patients. The aspiring writer's ability to bridge the gap between writing for examination and other purposes and writing a polished article for publication may be underestimated. Although there are some obvious differences between these two types of writing, they are not as great as might be thought. More importantly, even experienced writers rarely produce their end product at first attempt. Providing there is a willingness to write and refine the material three, four or more times, a polished and readable end product will emerge.

PUBLISHED MATERIALS

Most writers rely in some way on previously published materials. Chapters 6 and 7 discuss how these can be located, reviewed and incorporated into written work. Use can be made of previously published materials in various other ways. First, they show what a successfully written piece of work looks and feels like and how it is presented. Published materials represent a model from which to work. In using published work for this purpose the writer is able to examine how language is used (and misused), how the material is broken up by headings and subheadings, how diagrams, graphs and tables can enliven a text, and the means by which references are built into the publication.

If the material requires a summary, examination of a published article which includes one will be of help. If writing for a particular journal, scrutinizing articles that have recently appeared in it will provide a feel for the style and format of successful publications.

PEER-GROUP ASSISTANCE

The aspiring writer should discuss ideas with colleagues, who then serve as a microcosm of a potential readership to help clarify thoughts about the proposed paper. Having to explain ideas to another person considerably sharpens the mind. The writer should look for, and expect, support and encouragement from colleagues, particularly those in more senior positions. Indeed, bearing in mind the importance of literature to the development of every profession, all professionals have an explicit obligation to support, encourage and reward those of its members who are writing for publication.

After starting to write and develop a first draft, this should be shown to colleagues with a knowledge of the subject. Their help in reviewing the material has two important functions: to review its content as someone with a thorough knowledge of the subject and to provide feedback as a potential reader of the published article. If possible, early and subsequent drafts of the work should be shown to a colleague who has publishing experience.

LIBRARIES AND LIBRARIANS

In constructing any piece of material for publication it is necessary to either read around the subject informally or undertake a formal literature review as part of its construction. In either event access to one or more professional libraries and specialist librarians is essential. At a local level such libraries might include those at the colleges and universities that offer courses in health care. In general there is generous access to a range of local library facilities and their invariably helpful and co-operative staff. Many local libraries participate in the inter-library loans scheme which enables members to borrow from other libraries; this service may or may not be free.

Access to regional and national libraries is also available, some providing specialist bibliographies and general and specific advice in addition to lending the usual library materials. Although staff in some such libraries prefer to be contacted by letter, many can be reached by telephone to discuss particular requirements. Libraries and their staff are extremely important resources for all writers. In particular, the assistance and advice from experienced librarians, many of whom have a thorough understanding of the professional literature, will be most valuable. Librarians are very willing to give assistance, particularly to beginners who are unsure about how to find their way around the library. (See also Chapter 6, 'Literature Search'.)

PUBLISHERS

The basic sequence of events in writing for publication is that the writer writes, the publisher publishes and the reader reads. The publisher, as intermediary between writer and reader, has a key role to play in maximizing the skill of the writer. Publishers, or more usually their editors, are accessible and most helpful in giving advice and support to writers.

Journals contain details of the editor and editorial staff, including work address and telephone numbers. The writer should contact the editor as an idea is developing in order to discuss it and to get and make use of advice based on considerable experience. Editors are more able to assist if they get more rather than less written information about the proposed paper. Whilst it would be acceptable to write to a publisher and ask if they would be interested in a paper describing a specific clinical technique, it would be more appropriate to ask the same question of the editor and to include an outline of the proposed paper that will enable them to assess the possibilities of the proposal.

Advice about the general requirements and style of articles and books can be obtained from publishers and editors; they are in the business of publishing and cannot do so unless writers write. They are eager to encourage and help writers, particularly beginners, and should be regarded as a resource to which there is full and free access. These topics are covered in more detail in Chapters 10 and 15.

TYPIST

Although all the preliminary work may be done in pencil on one side of the paper with very large margins and spaces for corrections, the final product should be typewritten. This applies to virtually all examples of writing, with the possible exception of examination work, and may be an absolute requirement for some items such as theses and works for publication. Unless the writer has the appropriate typing skills it is as well to employ a professional typist to do the job. They can usually be obtained from a local agency or, more frequently, by asking around the secretarial staff in the writer's place of work and hiring a typist to do the job privately. There is no doubt that well-typed material and the assistance of a good typist are a very valuable resource.

Some employers, educational institutions for example, provide their staff with access to word processors. Alternatively, many writers prefer to invest a modest sum of money in a word processor in order to be able to do the job personally. (See Chapter 21, 'Writing Technology'.)

VISUAL AIDS

On occasion it might be necessary to reproduce material in forms other than the written word. If simple graphs, tables or charts are to be used, the author might be able to do this personally. However, if other forms of artwork are necessary, the audio-visual aids, printing or photographic departments in the workplace should be contacted for advice and assistance. This resource might have to be paid for but the cost is usually reasonable. If it is anticipated that these services will be necessary, requirements should be discussed with the appropriate staff as soon as possible. It is obviously important that any use of illustrative materials be discussed with the prospective publisher.

Writers are thus not confined only to the use of written words. The use of other forms of presentation is always worth serious consideration. (See Chapter 8, 'Illustrations'.)

REFERENCE BOOKS

A number of reference books are of use in relation to writing. They include a dictionary, a thesaurus and books such as this one which are designed for those developing their writing skills. In addition, some publishers may refer writers to specialist publications that deal with indexing, writing style and the use of references. A number of such texts are contained in the 'Recommended Reference Texts' at the end of this book.

SELF-HELP GROUPS

Writing for publication, and the development of writing skills, need not necessarily be a solitary activity. This is particularly so if there are others in the locality, from any of the health care professions, who also wish to develop this skill. Examples of how such a common aim might be achieved are by organizing a writing workshop and a journal club which includes critical evaluation of writers' style and article structure.

THE SOCIETY OF AUTHORS

In return for a membership fee the Society of Authors provides book authors with a range of services which include advising on contract negotiation and on how to take up complaints on any issue concerned with authorship. The address is: The Society of Authors, 84 Drayton Gardens, London SW10 9SB.

AUTHOR'S AGENT

An agent may be employed to negotiate a book contract with a potential publisher. Apart from advising on the detail of all contract clauses, an important function of the agent is to negotiate a favourable contract generally, and royalty payments in particular. The Society of Authors produces a guide on authors' agents.

The aspiring author should *never* struggle on alone in the mistaken belief that use should not be made of the many resources which are available. All those described here, and others, are there to be fully utilized by the beginning and experienced writer.

Chapter 4
Writing Style and Structure

Attention to writing style and structure improves the quality and readability of written work. Although writing is a very individual skill and no absolute rules exist to cover every situation, there are a few general points which help in developing style and structure. A clearly written paper is more likely to be produced if consideration is given to planning, structure and content of the paper before it is written.

PLANNING

Planning begins with the advancement of often vague ideas which will form the subject of the paper. At each subsequent phase as it progresses from vague ideas to a complete paper, planning makes production of the paper that much easier. This phase, which applies equally to a piece of coursework, a dissertation or an item for publication, is a crucial part of the writing process.

There is no doubt that the longer an idea is given to mature and evolve, the easier it is to get it on paper. Although there is a need to be careful about spending too much time 'thinking it over', some time must be given to considering the subject before putting pen to paper. A colleague of mine who is an excellent thinker and writer uses the time spent on long motor-car journeys to develop ideas and for constructing the outline of an article, and is then ready to write an excellent first draft. Although few have that type of ability, thinking time given to the planning of material in advance of writing is time well spent.

During this thinking time, it is important to make rough notes, for example general headings with brief explanations, which will form the skeleton of the written material. These notes may initially appear unimportant but they can be of much assistance when thought is being given to the structure of the paper.

During the planning stage the requirements of the publisher, or of the institution or person who will examine the work, must be obtained and studied. The aspiring writer needs to be clear about what is required, for example in terms of length and style.

STRUCTURE

The structure and shape of the work needs to be considered, and notes made as tentative decisions are taken. At least three separate but related items are considered here: sections, the order of sections, and their size.

Sections

The material is broken into sections of appropriate length. Examples are chapters in books, major parts in articles, and paragraphs within an article. Although there are few firm rules concerning how an item should be written and broken into sections, the subject is of considerable importance. The number of headings, subheadings, sub-subheadings and sub-sub-subheadings will depend on the length and complexity of the paper.

It is usual to indicate the beginning and end of sections by using headings, subheadings and sub-subheadings of differing styles and location within the body of the text. It is important to establish clearly the hierarchy required. This will be reflected by the publisher in the final design of the book. Apart from consistency, there are no firm rules regarding the style and location of headings. The following example would be quite adequate:

MAJOR HEADING	(capital letters, centred)
A Subheading	(first letter of each word in capital letters, centred)
A sub-subheading	(first letter in capital letters, not centred)

An aid to making decisions regarding this aspect of structure is to examine published works, paying particular attention to how they are broken into major and minor sections. These represent successes which have been scrutinized by writers and editors. When the work is given to colleagues for review, it is also advisable to ask for comment on section length and position.

Order of sections

The order and sequence of the main sections must be planned in advance of writing. Although most writers are clear about the first, middle and last sections of the paper, that is, the introduction, body and conclusion, other parts present an additional challenge. There are two possible ways of reducing this difficulty. The first is to examine the proposed structure and look for a logical sequence of sections, each being placed in relation to others because a positive decision has been made with regard to its placement. Example 1 shows what the structure of a research report might look like.

Example 1 _____

Structure of a research report

    Part 1   Introduction

    Part 2   Literature review

    Part 3   Research method

    Part 4   Pilot study

    Part 5   Main study

    Part 6   Data analysis

    Part 7   General discussion and conclusions

For some works a structure may have to be developed for that specific purpose. For example, if a clinician is preparing an article describing the development of a new case conference method, it might have the structure illustrated in Example 2.

Example 2 _____

Structure of an article

    Part 1   Case conference structure. Definition and description

    Part 2   Historical development of the case conference

    Part 3   Elements of the case conference

    Part 4   Case conference participants

    Part 5   Case conference documentation

    Part 6   Chairing the case conference

    Part 7   Discussion, problems and plans for the future

Providing that time and consideration are given to the sequence of sections, there should be few problems. All that is required is that every item and section appears, in relation to other items and sections, as a result of a conscious decision. Nothing should be left to chance.

Size of sections

The size of different parts of a piece of written work is an individual decision, but attention must be given as soon as possible to the length of each part. A section with the same title, 'Literature Review' for example, may constitute very different proportions of the total length of two different pieces of written work. For example, in a coursework essay a section entitled 'Literature Review' may attract 10% of the total marks. Bearing in mind that many such essays have a stipulated maximum length, it would be inappropriate to devote 90% of the total essay length to reviewing the literature. However, it might be realistic to devote 10% of the length to such a review. By contrast an article intended to review the literature on a particular subject may appropriately devote 90% of its length to this topic.

CONTENT

The content of a paper is predetermined by the choice of subject matter. *Only* the chosen subject and related material must be included. It is for the writer to decide what to include and exclude. Again, conscious and deliberate decisions must be made. If items of peripheral importance are deliberately included, that will have to be explained.

The point of writing is to convey ideas to the reader in a way which is to the point, is clear and is as attractively written as possible. Considerable effort must be made to exclude irrelevant material. When the paper is complete, the writer should scrutinize each part and ask: 'Do I really want to include this, and would the quality of the paper be reduced if it were omitted?'. Clear, readable work will be easier to produce if the question 'Is this *really* what I want to say?' is asked frequently.

Many works contain a mixture of fact and opinion. It is necessary to ensure that these are not confused in the mind of the reader. Ideally, sections containing fact should be separated from those containing opinion. If this is not possible, then the writer must ensure that readers are informed what is fact and what is opinion. This can be done by presenting facts using such wording as 'With the majority of patients it is possible and desirable to reduce post-operative pain significantly'. Opinions may be expressed in the following form: 'In my opinion, the quality of health care is gradually improving'.

WRITING

Having planned the material and made decisions about the structure and content, the serious writing now starts. The writer should begin as soon as possible, anticipating that a number of drafts will be necessary before the final stage is reached. The use of jargon, repetition and ambiguous statements should be avoided and can be edited out as further drafts are written. Rough notes are converted into a first and subsequent drafts. Each draft should be read aloud so that it is possible to hear the flow of words, and colleagues should be asked to review the various drafts. It is extremely rare for a first or second draft to be the final one.

For all but the final draft the choice of writing material and approach are a matter of personal choice. For example using a pencil on one side of the paper, leaving wide margins and large spaces between sections, might help redrafting. The use of a word processor makes rewriting very easy. The previously prepared plan relating to the structure and content must now be filled out. The amount of words allocated to each part of the work must be used in relation to each heading, subheading and so on.

It is more usual to write the parts of the paper in the same sequence as will be found in the final draft, but this is not always so or necessary. If it is easier to write a middle or end part before writing the earlier one, the writer should do so. Writing out of sequence is better than waiting a long time for the inspiration to get started on the first part of the paper. All that needs to be done here is to write the different parts of the paper on their own pages and subsequently rearranged them in the correct order. Again, the use of a word processor makes this easy. If this approach is used for a long piece of work such as a book or a research report, it is as well to number the pages with chapter and page numbers. For example, pages of Chapter 4 should be marked 4.1, 4.2, 4.3, 4.4 and so on.

ASPECTS OF STYLE

Although writing style is not the principal concern of this book, that being left to the authors of publications in the 'Recommended Reference Texts', a few key areas will be discussed. They have been selected because they are in common use and because they can cause beginning writers some difficulty which is relatively easy to resolve.

Words should be short, sharp, meaningful and easily understood. Each needs careful selection and placement within the sentence. A good dictionary should be consulted if there is any uncertainty about exact meaning or spelling. Where possible, a variety of words with the same meaning should be used to avoid repetition; a thesaurus can be consulted for alternatives. Repetition can, and should, be used intentionally as a means of emphasizing an important point or for dramatic effect. Neither a thesaurus nor a dictionary should be used to find a longer or more impressive word.

Sentences should be neither too long nor too short. Readers want to grasp the meaning of the sentence without having to reread it or first break it into its component parts.

A *paragraph* is a group of sentences (occasionally just one) in which a single topic is presented. If the paragraph is becoming too long, in excess of 200 words for example, it is necessary to consider whether the material is really only dealing with one topic.

Quotation marks (sometimes referred to as inverted commas) are used in writing mainly to designate the beginning and end of words or sentences which are being quoted directly from the work of others. There are several types, but the two most commonly used in Western literature are: single, '. . .' and double, ". . .". British printers adhere to the use of the former whereas American printers tend to employ the latter. Placement of punctuation outside or inside the closing quotation mark also varies between countries. For work not to be published, it is sufficient to use common sense and consistent application. Quotation marks are also used to draw attention to words used in an unusual context: slang or colloquialisms for example.

Italics are a useful method of emphasizing a word or group of words. They are the writer's equivalent of the speaker's spoken emphasis: for example: 'We *must* win'. Underlining to indicate emphasis is used in both handwritten and typewritten material. Printers, unless instructed to do otherwise, will set all underlined items in italics. Underlining to be retained as in an equation is identified as a 'rule', and an encircled marginal note to that effect should be added to indicate what is required. Italic type is used formally to indicate book and journal titles and also to identify foreign words other than those in common use in the language in which the author is writing. In English, for example, words such as 'via' and 'petite' would not be italicized.

Listing, with letters or numbers, is used when it is essential that the items be shown or displayed in a one, two, three or A, B, C format. The technique is one that can easily be overused and abused so that it intrudes into the presentation of ideas.

Parentheses, or round brackets, are an integral part of a commonly used reference system: 'Jones (1993) suggested that . . .' is an example. Parentheses are also used to separate a distantly connected idea within a statement, where the writer wishes to elaborate or explain further or digress slightly from the main theme of the sentence as in a parenthetical remark. The more closely connected idea would be shown between commas and dashes. As with the overuse of listing, quotation marks and abbreviations, the too frequent use of parentheses can be intrusive and distracting.

Brackets, or square brackets, are used to insert the writer's words or correction within a direct quotation from another published work, as in 'When they [the writers] set pen to papre [*sic*] the printers . . .'. The term '[*sic*]' indicates that the quoted passage, which is shown exactly as in the original contains an error. If permissible, it is often kinder to avoid the latter use and simply correct an obvious typographical error; perpetuating an innocent literal serves no purpose, especially to the source author. Brackets in varying shapes are also used in mathematical expressions.

Abbreviations are necessary in some forms of writing, but run the risk of overuse in others. For example, if frequent reference is made in the text to the National Health Service, it should be written in full the first time it appears followed by its abbreviated form in parentheses: (NHS). Thereafter, the abbreviation may be used in place of the full title: NHS without the parentheses.

Abbreviations such as i.e., e.g. and etc. are probably best written in full, if for no other reason than to stimulate the choice of alternatives and, more importantly, to avoid their overuse. One occasion when the abbreviated use of words is always used as 'et al.'. This is an abbreviation for the Latin words et alii which mean 'and others'. When referring to three or more joint authors of a reference used in the text, the names of them all can be given on the first occasion. Thereafter the name of the first author is given, followed by 'et al.' Thus, 'Clark, Fitzpatrick and Jones' becomes 'Clark et al.' in subsequent citations. Although this convention is used in the text, it should never be used in a list of references; there all names must be presented. There is a full stop after et al.

Ellipses are used to indicate that material has been omitted from a sentence or paragraph, by a writer who is quoting from another's work. The resultant abbreviated quotation can still be understood, the ellipses indicating that an undisclosed amount of redundant material has been removed without changing the meaning of the original work. Thus, 'Please, if I might be so bold, may I help you?' might become 'Please . . . may I help you?' The omitted words are indicated by the use of three points, . . ., inserted in the middle of the sentence where words have been removed; if the omission occurs at the end of a sentence, there is a fourth point or other appropriate closing punctuation. In fairness to readers it is necessary to ensure that the selected part of the sentence conveys the meaning intended by the original writer.

Capital letters are always used at the beginning of proper nouns: New York and James, for example. Confusion sometimes arises when using terms such as general wards or departments in hospitals, or in an informal reference to the college, university or operating theatre. As these are nouns rather than proper nouns, they do not require capital letters. For titles of literary works such as books, plays, journals, articles and poems, each major word may begin with a capital letter, or only the first word might have one. Thus an article title might read 'The Development of Health Care' or 'The development of health care'. Whichever convention is used, the only requirement is that it be consistently used throughout the text.

Gender use in the form of he/she and him/her may need special consideration, particularly when the terms are used often. For example in many textbooks, authors state early in the text that staff will be referred to as 'she' and the patient/client as 'he'. This convention is quite common and avoids the alternative reference to staff as he/she, and to patient/client as he/she. Additionally, the consistent use of 'she' for staff and 'he' for patient/client (or the reverse) helps the reader to recognize which of the two groups is being referred to.

In those instances when it is felt that specific gender is inappropriate, he/she and him/her is acceptable.

A third alternative and nowadays the one most widely preferred is to write in such a way that the terms he, she, him and her are not generally used. Although this approach requires a more careful choice of words it can be done. Consider this passage which makes no attempt to avoid gender identification.

> My wife is a doctor, having been one for five years. My son and daughter are also doctors; there are now three in the family. When I first asked a colleague why medicine was such a popular career, she replied that 'working with people' might be an important factor.

The same passage, rewritten to avoid gender use might read:

> My spouse is a doctor, having been one for five years. My two children are also doctors; there are now three in the family. When I first asked a colleague why medicine was such a popular career, the reply indicated that 'working with people' might be an important factor.

Once a decision has been made about which gender style to use, this must be followed. It is worth checking with the publisher for their house style.

If the work is not being published, careful reading by the writer and a friend will minimize potential problems. If it is being published, problems can also be ironed out as the manuscript goes through its various draft stages. Although publishers obviously prefer to receive a manuscript which is well developed in terms of style, structure, presentation and grammar, they will also be helpful and considerate if it has some rough edges. Publishers will *not* reject good ideas because the manuscript is poorly presented. Rather, they will encourage and help the writer to improve the paper. However, any publisher will stress to authors that changes *cannot* be made after typesetting has commenced. This is because of the high cost of making corrections at proof stage.

GENERAL GUIDELINES FOR EFFECTIVE WRITING

Effective writing is being able to convey, using a minimum of words, ideas and information to the reader in a way which is clear and readable. The following general guidelines, which are not in any order of priority, are offered as aids to the beginner.

- The aspiring author must become familiar with the subject *before* starting to write. Even the specialist in the subject should try to improve knowledge of it by further reading. See Chapters 6 and 7 which deal with searching and reviewing the literature.

- Thoughts must be organized on paper and consideration must be given to the structure and sequence of the parts of the work. It should not be assumed that the best possible sequence will emerge without careful and deliberate planning.
- It is necessary to ensure that the material is written to meet the requirements of the examiner, reader or publisher. The writer must become familiar with the marking criteria if the material is to be examined, and with the style and general requirements of the editor if the work is to be published.
- It is important to write clearly and briefly, demonstrating a good command of the language in which the paper is written. Simply written and easily read material reflects a high level of writing skill and a thorough understanding of the subject.
- The overuse of lists and abbreviations such as e.g., etc., and i.e. should be avoided. Lists can be minimized by the appropriate use of sentences in the form of prose, and abbreviations by the use of the word or term.
- The writer should not strive for perfection in the earlier drafts of a paper.
- It is important to be prudent in the use of references to published materials. Overuse can be as much of a problem as underuse. If the work is to be published, the writer must ensure that the reference system used meets the requirements of the journal or publishing house.
- A firm timetable should be set for completing the work by deciding to write a specific number of words in a given time, for example a 1000-word first draft of a paper over a one-week period.
- It is important to be critical of work as it is produced. One or more colleagues should be asked to critically review it by commenting on the successful and less successful parts of the paper.

Chapter 5
References

Whether or not written material is to be published, it is likely that formal references to previously published work will be included; one possible exception is written material prepared under examination conditions without access to notes, books and so on.

The term *reference* relates to the bibliographical description of author, title and other features of a published work. The inclusion of a formal reference has only one purpose: to direct the reader to it. For example, if reference is made to a work by Black (1992), sufficient bibliographical detail must be given to enable the reader to find that publication.

The term *publication* is used to describe any idea or information which is made available to others by means of the written word, which may be a formally published work or a privately distributed piece of writing, or something 'published' verbally at a conference. The term also includes forthcoming publications such as those that have been accepted, but not yet published, by a journal. If the material being referred to has not yet been actually published (an unpublished paper or a conference presentation, for example), the author of the work must be contacted personally and permission sought to refer to it. An exact copy of the item of unpublished material to be referred to must be sent to the original author for approval. This gives the author an opportunity to check that he or she has been correctly interpreted and quoted. This requirement does not apply to the inclusion of references to actually published materials such as articles, books and other publications. If, however, extensive portions of published material are to be used, or illustrations published by someone else, permission must be requested from the author and/or the publisher, or whoever holds the copyright. If in doubt, it is vital that permission be sought.

Example 3 incorporates the details that would be included when seeking permission to reproduce a lengthy block of text or illustrations from a copyright holder.

USE OF REFERENCES

When writing for a professional readership, writers invariably make references to already published works. A list of those references used in

Example 3 _____

Permission letter

1 Cottage Close
Kearnsly
Lancs LC1 GD4
4 July 1993

Permissions Editor
Smart Publications
14 Fort Place
Dulforth DD2 6HG

Dear Sir/Madam,

In my forthcoming book *Writing for Health Care Professions*, to be published by Blackwell Scientific Publications in 1993, I would like to include the following material from Purple, M. (1989) *Health Care in Europe:*

pages 14–15 Table 5, and page 98 Figure 7
    and
page 195, from 4th line 'The future of health care...' to page 196, midway through final paragraph '... early in the next century.'

I would be grateful if you would grant me permission to use the material specified above. Appropriate acknowledgement will, of course, be made.

I enclose a self-addressed and stamped envelope for return of the attached permission slip.

Yours sincerely

Desmond F.S. Cormack

. . . .

Permission is hereby granted to Desmond F.S. Cormack to incorporate the above-specified material from Purple, M. (1989) *Health Care in Europe* into his forthcoming book *Writing for Health Care Professions* to be published by Blackwell Scientific Publications.

Signed. . . . .

Permissions Editor, Smart Publications

Date. . . . .

the text is placed at the end of the piece of coursework or of the thesis, article, chapter or book, for example. While this is the case generally, there are exceptions and not every work will include references; for example a book review or a letter to the editor of a professional journal may or may not include them. Although the basic function of the inclusion of full bibliographical references is to direct the reader to the materials referred to, the reason for their initial inclusion in the text must be considered. The major reasons for including reference materials are to support one's views and to inform.

Irrespective of the topic written about, most authors realize that their knowledge of the subject is much more limited than they at first thought. It is therefore prudent to learn about the subject by reading what others have written about it before starting to write. This approach is neither new nor unusual in that most writers and students will look for ideas, knowledge and inspiration from the written work of others. It is not being suggested that a writer simply repeat what has been read. However, old ideas and existing knowledge, added to the author's personal ideas and knowledge, can result in a better contribution to the literature. In short, there is no point in 're-inventing the wheel'; the job of the writer is to be aware of existing knowledge and to add to it.

Learning about the subject by reading published works is of particular importance to those undertaking a piece of research. For example, the researcher will wish to read relevant materials relating to the methods and findings of research in similar areas.

In undertaking any piece of research it is vital that the researcher, who will subsequently become the writer of the research report, be fully aware of pre-existing literature. The research report will contain full references to all the literature that was read and incorporated into the research project.

The citation by the writer of relevant and valuable references helps readers to extend their own knowledge of the subject.

SYSTEMS OF CITATION

In professional works the two most commonly used methods of citing references, that is, of incorporating them into a paper, are the Harvard and numerical systems.

Harvard system

The most widely used system is referred to as the Harvard system. It involves giving the surname of the author in the text, followed by the year of publication. Usually, both are enclosed in parentheses unless the author's name is part of the sentence. Such reference citations might read:

The development of a positive relationship between the clinician and patient is regarded as being essential to the provision of high quality care (Jones 1991). This view was supported in a subsequent paper by Smith (1992).

When using the Harvard system it is important to remember that, apart from the ideas and information expressed by the writer being cited, *only* the surname of the author and year of publication are included in the text as a reference label. At the end of the article or other work a list containing full bibliographical details of all the references cited in the text will appear. The title of the list will be the single word *References*, beneath which will be an alphabetically arranged list of references. Although the presentation of book references will be slightly different from that of journal references, there are a number of similarities (see Example 4).

Example 4 _____

Harvard reference system

The relationship between the ratio of trained to untrained staff and the quality of care given to hospitalized patients has been commented on by a number of writers including Black (1989), White (1990) and Green (1992). In a paper by Scarlett (1985) this relationship is described as being: '... positive, in that the greater the ratio of trained to untrained staff, the better the quality of care' (p. 4).

A rather more constrained view was expressed by Brown (1986) who suggested that an increase in the ratio of trained to untrained staff *may* result in improved care. Mustard (1990), who suggested that far too little was known about the subject, recommended that it urgently required researching. Much earlier, a similar view was expressed by Blue, Black and White (1980) but was never acted on. Blue *et al.* also produced one of the earliest computer-based manpower planning packages.

REFERENCES

Black, F. (1989) *Staffing in Health Care*. London, Clarkson.
Blue, D., Black, S. and White, H. (1980) *Calculating Establishments in the Health Care Professions*. Chicago, Firth Publications.
Brown, M. (1986) *Politics and Health Economics*. Edinburgh, Johnston.
Green, K. (1992) Paramedical costs and cost benefits. *Health Care Management*, **23**, 67–9.
Mustard, B. (1990) Staffing issues. In Pink, N. (ed.) *Care and Care Issues*, pp. 234–43. London, Gladstone.
Scarlett, D. (1985) Inputs and outcomes. *International Journal of Hospital Administration*, **32**, 118–24.
White, T. (1990) Trained–Untrained Staff Ratios. Doctor of Philosophy thesis, University of Newtown.

Multiple authorship

When using the Harvard system and referring to three or more joint authors of a reference used in the text, the names of them all can be given on the first occasion. Thereafter the name of the first author followed by *et al.* is given. Thus, Blue, Black and White becomes Blue *et al.* Although this convention is used in the text, it must never be used in the reference list, where all names must be presented.

The numerical system

The numerical system (also known as the Vancouver system) can take one of two forms. First, publications cited (referred to) in the text are numbered as they appear in sequence. At each point in the text where information from another published source is cited, its number is inserted in parentheses or as a superscript. The text might appear as: 'In a more recent paper (1) it was shown that . . .'.

Alternatively the second form of numerical system can include the surname of the author and a sequential number. The text might appear as: 'In a more recent paper, Jones (1) showed that . . .'. In either event, the references are subsequently listed in numerical order.

If different parts of a published piece are referred to in the text, the appropriate page numbers may be added to the text in addition to the reference. For instance, 'In a more recent paper (1, p. 12) it was shown that . . .'.

At the end of text that uses the numerical system, the references appear under the heading 'References' but are listed in numerical sequence instead of alphabetically (see Example 5).

Example 5

Numerical reference system

The frequency with which the economics of clinical issues is being discussed in the literature has increased manyfold in recent years (1). According to some authorities this trend will continue well into the next century as computer systems are developed which will enable individual clinical activities to be accurately costed (2–4).

REFERENCES

1. Black, J. (1987) *The National Health Service*, Manchester, Health Publications Ltd.
2. White, F. (1992) The cost of care. *Health Service Personnel*, **5**, 4–10.
3. Green, P. (1993) Computing care costs. *Health Care Computing*, **67**, 34–6.
4. Blue, V. (1992) *The Economics of Health Care*. Toronto, Tropper Publications.

Book references

Irrespective of the system used, references to books and journals are treated identically within the text. However, they are handled differently in the reference list.

A reference to a book must contain the surname and initial(s) of the first name(s) of the author or editor, the year of publication in parentheses, the title of the book (which when underlined by the writer indicates to the printer that italics must be used), the edition of the book which is being referred to if more than one edition has been published, the city of publication and the name of the publisher. Example 6 illustrates an acceptable style for presenting a book reference. The title of the book (underlined in the manuscript and therefore set in italics by the printer) shows initial capitalization of the first word and of all the major words that follow.

Example 6 _____

Book reference

Jones, T. (1992) *Health and Happiness*. London, Professional
Publications.

Article references

A reference to a journal article also must contain the author's name, the year of publication, the title of the article, the name of the journal (underlined) in which the article appeared, the volume number of the journal (with the issue number in brackets), and the first and last page numbers of the article. Example 7 shows how a reference to an article can be presented. The convention is to capitalize the first letter of the article title and the first letter of any proper names following, and to underline the journal title.

Example 7 _____

Article reference

Black, H. (1992) Care and the influence of economics. *The British Journal
of Health Economics*, **5**, 67–73.

Unpublished reference (unpublished paper or conference presentation)

A reference to an unpublished paper, included only with the written permission of its author, will enable the reader of the reference to locate the original publication directly or through its author. A reference to an unpublished (written) paper should follow the format of Example 8.

Example 8 ───────────────────────────────────

Reference to an unpublished paper

Black, G. (1992) *The application of psychological principles to health care issues.* Unpublished paper. Regional Psychology Unit, District General Hospital, London.

───

A reference to an unpublished paper which had been read at a conference should follow the format of Example 9.

Example 9 ───────────────────────────────────

Reference to a conference paper

White, L. (1991) *A healthy elderly population: An aim of total health care.* Unpublished paper. Opening address at National Health Care Conference, 18 July 1992. Association of Health Care Managers, London.

───

BIBLIOGRAPHY

A bibliography is a list of references relating to a specific subject such as 'Multidisciplinary teamwork', or 'The function of the case conference', or 'Informed consent in clinical research'. A bibliography may be constructed by someone who is interested in or researching a specific subject, who is writing about a topic, or who is a student of the subject. The list of references of which a bibliography is composed is presented in alphabetical order.

A number of libraries provide bibliographies on various subject areas on request. Whatever the professional subject of the required bibliography, it is worth while asking local and national professional libraries whether they have one.

A common error made in relation to a bibliography is to confuse it with the list of references cited in a text, which appears at the end of written works. It will be remembered that a reference list is a list of references that are cited, or referred to, in a text and which appear in a list at the end of the text under the heading 'References'. A referenced piece of work may also have a bibliography in addition to the list of references. Whereas all items in the reference list will have been referred to in the text, none of the items in the bibliography (if there is one) will have been referred to in the text. Thus, items in the bibliography relate to the subject of the text, but are in addition to those references used in the text and subsequently contained in the reference list.

Annotated bibliography

A bibliography is a collection of references relating to a specific topic: pain or anxiety, for example. An *annotated bibliography* is one in which each of the references is accompanied by a critical or explanatory note. Producing an annotated bibliography is a particularly useful exercise in relation to coursework preparation. For example a student may be requested to write an essay on a given subject, make appropriate references to published literature *and* produce an annotated bibliography of a given length. An example of one annotated item (reference) in a bibliography is given in Example 10.

Example 10

Annotated bibliography: Care in the community

Violet, D. (1991) Who looks after the elderly with multiple pathology? *Journal of Community Care*, **5**, 89–94.

This paper, which is research based, is written by a physiotherapist, nurse, general practitioner and social worker. Research data were collected from a 10% sample of all people aged 65 years or more in an industrial town (population 39 000) in northern England. The response rate was 87%. The aim of the study was to describe the quantity and type of care provided by all professional and voluntary agencies, and by relatives and other informal carers. This well written paper is convincing, contains valuable research-based clinical data, identifies gaps in service provision, and recommends strategies for the future.

GENERAL GUIDELINES FOR USING REFERENCEES

- The writer must ensure that the method of using and writing references meets the requirements of the person who will examine or publish the work being written. If these requirements are not made known, it is necessary to ask for them.
- A formal and acceptable method of citation, such as the Harvard or numerical system, must be used for presentation of references. It is important to be consistent in the use of references and to employ one system throughout. There are two common methods of citing references within the text. They are quoting and paraphrasing.

Direct quotations may be presented as:

'In recent years there has been a considerable increase in the expectations of the public in relation to their quality of care' (Black 1992, p. 23).

In paraphrasing, writers use their own words to describe the idea or information contained in all or part of the text being referred to. For example:

> From the 1980s onwards the public have become much more demanding in terms of seeking high quality care. (See Black 1992, p. 23.)

With experience, the ability to vary the ways and phrases used to incorporate references into the text can be developed. Clearly it would be boring if an otherwise quite appropriate phrase such as 'According to . . .' was used repetitively. Variations in the introductory phrase include: 'It was suggested by . . .', 'In the opinion of . . .', 'An alternative view was expressed by . . .' and 'Black expressed it thus . . .'.

- The overuse of reference materials is as much a writing fault as is underuse. Indeed, it is common for published works to be so laden with references as to intrude upon the clarity of the writer's ideas and to make the work tedious to read. The exception to this rule is the review article in which the writer does little other than review and evaluate published works.

- As a general rule references are required when the idea, statement or knowledge being used is not universally accepted and when the material can be attributed to one or more writers. For example, if a writer made a general statement to the effect that senile dementia was age related, it would not be necessary to provide a reference. However, if the writer wished to state the exact relationship between age and senile dementia in terms of the percentage of a given population who would develop the illness, then use of a reference would be appropriate.

- When collecting references, whether for a project or for publication, it is useful to keep some information about them, for example on 10 cm × 15 cm (4 in × 6 in) filing cards which can be stored in an alphabetical index system, usually under the first letter of the author's surname. The card should contain the formal reference to the publication, the library or some other place where the material can be obtained, and brief details of the content of the reference material.

- The ability to use references is an integral part of professional writing generally, and of writing for publication in particular. Although the majority of beginning writers have little experience of using references in a formal way, the skill can easily be learned. Many beginners successfully develop this technique quickly, and others 'get the hang of it' within a few days of being introduced to the topic.

Chapter 6
Literature Search

Literature searching is an essential skill in the production of any professional paper. The professional knowledge captured in the written word of predecessors provides a base from which thinking, practice and skills can be advanced or challenged. However, such is the volume of material now available that without the skills to identify, locate and sort this rich source much valuable time and effort can be wasted. This chapter discusses the various sources of literature and how they can be located and searched.

PROFESSIONAL LITERATURE

Professional literature comes in many formats. The majority is still produced as paper publications, but electronic or microfiche media are increasingly being used. Literature can be generated by individuals, groups, academic institutions, professional organizations, government departments, and manufacturers and suppliers of products. Irrespective of the medium or the source, the volume of material available to health professionals is such that, unless there is an effective and efficient way of identifying only those materials that are of direct relevance to the area of interest, an inordinate amount of time can be wasted skimming through the various sources. Not all sources deal with the same sort of material, and by understanding the characteristics of the various formats this will assist the user to be selective in assessing the literature. Example 11 lists the common formats used to publish professional literature.

Example 11 ————————————————————————

Common formats used to publish professional literature

Journals
Books
Reports
Theses
Conference proceedings
Government circulars
Computer databases
Microfiche

Journals

There is a vast selection of journals available, and there are two main types, primary and secondary.

Primary journals are those that publish original research and papers that have not been published elsewhere or in an alternative form. Papers published in primary journals are invariably refereed, that is, they have been examined by an independent external expert prior to publication. This ensures that the papers published meet a minimum professional and scholarly standard. Journals such as *The Lancet*, *Journal of Advanced Nursing*, *Social Science & Medicine* and *Quality Assurance in Health Care* are examples of primary sources.

Secondary journals do not usually publish original papers but can be a valuable source of information since it is common for these journals to publish a synopsis of original papers which appear in primary sources. This can be particularly useful since it gives the reader the opportunity to review what amounts to an abstract of the work which can then be followed up if desired. Secondary sources tend to publish material in a less technical, user-friendly format and often have appeal to a wider audience. Hence, secondary journals can be an ideal mechanism for disseminating work.

There are three main types of secondary journal: limited circulation, review and professional journals. Limited circulation journals tend to be produced and distributed free to members of organizations or special interest groups, for example *Lampada* which is distributed to Royal College of Nursing members. Review journals provide information on preselected topics often written by subject experts who will critically debate the findings or content of original work, for example *Geriatric Medicine Clinics*. Professional journals are aimed to cater for the needs of practitioners and will often address issues of knowledge utilization or changes in practice; an example is *Health Visitor*.

Although a clear distinction has been made between primary and secondary journals, the reality is that many primary journals will carry secondary synopses and similarly many secondary journals will publish original work. Indeed, some so-called secondary journals are refereed. This can be confusing and can result in the uninformed reader discounting a journal as a source of original and scholarly work on the basis of its apparent lineage.

Books

Much scholarly work is published in book format. In general the reader should expect a book to deal with a topic in much greater depth than that which appears in journal publications. In particular, books usually cover the previous literature published on the material in far greater detail.

Books can be by single authors or by groups of individuals working collectively, or are produced as a result of editing a number of independent but related papers which are integrated into a single text by an editor. Books that are the work of multiple authors often provide a higher standard of text since the individual chapters tend to be written by experts in the field. However, the editor needs to be skilful in ensuring that the separate contributions are well linked and complement one another, are consistent in style, of equal quality, and avoid unnecessary repetition of material. A poorly edited text can result in the converse. In addition, if a single theme is being progressed or advanced, this can be difficult to follow since the various authors may present arguments from slightly different perspectives.

Although new technology has advanced the rate with which books can be prepared, they will, on the whole, take a little longer to produce than getting material into print via the journal route. Hence, if a reader is interested in assessing the state of the science related to a particular field, it is probable that the most recent work will come from journals, conference proceedings, theses or limited distribution reports.

Reports

Reports can be a valuable source of information and a comparatively easy way to publish material if the target audience is relatively small. Many authors present reports that are essentially for use within an organization or that have a very limited circulation. The advantages are that with word processors, desktop publishers and high quality photocopy and binding equipment, material can be published quickly, with relative ease and at little cost. Material that is highly specialized and/or changes rapidly is often published in report format. The disadvantage of reports is that they are notoriously difficult to obtain or even know about unless the reader is part of the organization that has produced them. Some Regional Health Authorities and professional bodies endeavour to increase the availability of such publications by encouraging authors to submit copies of their work for abstracting and dissemination to other members. Original reports can often form the basis of subsequent publications in conference proceedings or journals. Despite this it can be useful and worth while to track down the original since it may contain greater detail, which for reasons of space, is omitted from published work. In particular it is common to find included within appendices of reports information on data collection instruments or other such valuable material.

Theses

When considering the latest developments in any field of science, no literature search is complete without reference to the product of higher academic study: dissertations and theses. The level of detail available in such publications can be impressive. Comprehensive and critical reviews of previous literature as well as detailed methodological sections are standard features of a high quality academic thesis which can provide a sound basis for further work. Unfortunately, there are usually only three or four copies of a thesis produced. However, the British Lending Library does keep copies on microfilm of all Doctoral and Master of Philosophy works completed in United Kingdom universities and central institutions. A similar service is available in the United States of America although in addition to PhD and MPhil work other doctoral degrees and masters programmes are covered.

Conference proceedings

Papers appearing in conference proceedings can provide a valuable source of information. Conference papers usually represent the cutting edge of thinking on a subject and often appear several months or even years before publication in scholarly journals or other more conventional forms. Although the material appearing in the written proceedings is often a summary of the full material presented at the conference, it is a worthwhile source and can provide a writer researching a topic with all the information necessary to contact the author for further details on the work described.

Government circulars

The Department of Health, the Management Executive and other governmental departments often publish papers and guidance that can address issues of major importance to a diverse group of health professionals. Whilst the better known reports attract considerable media interest, certain circulars are specifically targeted at professional groups and therefore may not be widely available. However, the Department of Health Library and Her Majesty's Stationery Office are usually very helpful in assisting a potential reader to track down material on a particular topic.

Computer databases

Readily available and relatively inexpensive computer technology has resulted in increasing amounts of information being produced in electronic format. For example, when purchasing computer technology or software, it is usual to obtain updates of the user's handbook on computer disk.

Databases are particularly useful for information that changes regularly or is rapidly increasing in volume. For example, although there are manual versions of abstracting services such as *Index Medicus*, the computer version *Medline* is more flexible and up to date (for more details see subsequent sections of this chapter). Unfortunately, operational use of these systems is often expensive since it requires the correct equipment and usually the use of a telephone line. Consequently the company running the service may charge quite high fees for access.

Microfiche

For many publications microfiche format is an alternative to the more standard hard-copy paper medium. A microfiche can come either as a film or in small postcard-sized sheets of plastic material. The original information, from a hard copy or an electronic database, is transcribed on to the microfiche by a process similar to photography. Journals frequently provide microfiche versions which save considerable space and are not subject to the wear, tear and degeneration associated with paper. In addition high-volume materials such as the records of full reference details, publisher information and current costs of all books in print are distributed to bookshops via microfiche. Those who need access to theses or dissertations of any postgraduate work via the British Library usually receive this in microfilm format. The advantage of this medium is the robust nature of the material and the large volumes of data that can be stored in a small space. However, to read the material requires access to a microfiche reader, and availability in most libraries does limit the location where the medium can be used. Similarly, if a copy of a page or pages of the material is required, access to a special hard-copy unit, which is often less readily available, is necessary. It is therefore important to investigate fully the resources available if access to material stored in microfiche medium is envisaged.

SELECTING A LIBRARY

When preparing to write an article it is essential that ready access to all necessary preparatory reading is available. It is highly unlikely that all the material required will be close at hand. Therefore it will be necessary to draw upon the services of a well stocked library.

Not all libraries are the same. Some cover certain subjects but not others. Similarly some will offer specialist services but may limit their use or even charge for the privilege. Other libraries, especially those that form part of a university or college, may restrict non-students to reading rights only. In order to be able to select the appropriate facilities for their needs, writers should be aware of what is available at well equipped libraries.

Subject specialist librarians

Perhaps the most valuable asset available to any library user is access to subject specialist librarians. These are individuals who, in addition to being skilled librarians, also have a detailed and in-depth knowledge of a specialist subject area. They will often have a command of the subject that will enable them to direct a reader to all the relevant material or at least give guidance on where to look. They will certainly be able to save users considerable time. Unfortunately, subject specialist librarians tend only to be available at the larger libraries or those attached to academic institutions. Smaller libraries may, however, form networks of specialists, whereby they can tap into the skills of a colleague in a different library. It is always worthwhile asking if there is a subject specialist available.

Cataloguing systems

Although readers may be able to browse effectively through a couple of shelves, they will not be able to find their way round a large health sciences library without a sound understanding of the cataloguing system. Unless readers know how material is catalogued, where it is stored and in what format, hours or even days can be spent aimlessly wandering round some of the larger libraries. The help of the librarian should be sought. It must not be assumed that all libraries use the same system. Most libraries will publish a short guide to the resources available and how to use the catalogue. It is worth taking the time to read the guide. This can save most users many hours of almost blind searching. Most librarians are happy to give new readers a tour of the library to assist them to use the resources effectively. Some libraries even offer access to a personal stereo that will 'talk the user round' the building, taking the reader from point to point giving a full explanation of services and the location of facilities and even offering instructions on how to find material.

There are a number of cataloguing systems that are commonly used in health science libraries. The two most frequently used are the *Dewey Decimal Classification Scheme* and the *National Library of Medicine Classification Scheme*. The Dewey Decimal Classification Scheme uses a series of numeric digits to break down topics from the general to the specific. The National Library of Medicine Classification Scheme uses a combination of letters and numbers. All libraries that use such systems will keep an up-to-date record of their holdings by maintaining a manual card index system or a computer database. Irrespective of the approach used it is worth investing some time in becoming fully familiar with the system so as to maximize the chance of finding material when conducting a literature search.

Textbooks and journals

It has already been said that not all libraries are the same, nor do they all carry the same range of textbooks or journals. Readers must therefore select a library that focuses its holding on the areas that interest them. Some libraries are given considerable funds to update stock whereas others are not, and it is important that users scan the shelves to ascertain whether new books and/or new editions are available. For many readers, journal holdings are the resource that is of prime importance. Not only should there be a wide selection of journals available but ideally they should have been subscribed to for as long a period as possible. A good, customer- friendly library will have a system that will enable users to make suggestions for additions to both the book and journal holdings.

Reference texts

Most libraries will have a reference-only section. This will include material that is in heavy demand or that is essential to enable users of the library to find other material, for example indexes, abstracts and bibliographies. Reference material may be available on a variety of media other than paper, that is, audio-visual tapes, microfiche or, increasingly, on-line or compact disk-based media.

Inter-library loan services

Even the best resourced libraries cannot afford to stock everything that every possible user may wish to access at one time. It is therefore important that a library subscribes to an inter-library loan facility. Some libraries organize such a service locally or on the basis of similar interests; others subscribe to the British Library inter-library loan scheme. This latter service effectively gives a subscriber access to a book, journal or holding held by any other subscribing library anywhere in the United Kingdom or indeed abroad. Unfortunately many libraries now charge for such a service although some do offer a degree of subsidy or, more rarely, provide the service free. One word of caution: the service can mean considerable delays in obtaining material, so it is necessary to plan well in advance if an inter-library loan is required.

Photocopy facilities

When collecting material for researching an article, most authors require access to photocopying facilities at reasonable cost. Most libraries do offer such facilities but will levy a charge. In some cases coin or pre-paid card-operated machines will be available. It is however important to recognize that there are strict copyright laws dictating the amount of photocopying and the use that can be made of photocopies. The librarian will be able to offer guidance on this subject.

Microfiche and microfilm readers

If users are likely to need access to theses or dissertations, it is important to check that there is a microfiche and/or microfilm reader available. Preferably there should also be facilities to enable hard copies of material from the fiche or film to be made if required. Hard copy facilities are essential if the library stores back copies of journals in microfiche format.

Compact disk readers

More and more reference materials, especially indexes and abstracts, are being produced on CD-ROM (compact disk read only memory) format. The availability of such technology indicates that the library is well advanced in its thinking about facilitating flexible access to material. The advantages of CD-ROM searching are discussed in more detail later in this chapter.

SEARCHING LITERATURE

Although a haphazard browse through the shelves or a flick through a few journals may yield a few articles of interest, such an approach would not adequately prepare a user to develop a tightly argued scholarly paper. If a comprehensive review of the literature on a specific subject is to be produced, the writer must go about the process in a systematic manner by searching the literature against predetermined criteria. Such a search can be conducted by either manual or computer methods and will need to draw on various tools, for example the subject index, author and classification catalogues, printed indexes, abstracts and bibliographies.

Subject index, author and classification catalogues

To enable libraries to keep track of their holdings and to enable users to find material, all libraries have subject indexes and author and classification catalogues covering their entire stock. A subject index can be thought of as an atlas to the library holdings. It provides the user with a breakdown of all the major and minor categories of material along with their associated classification codes and their location within the library. Author catalogues are simply an alphabetical listing of the holdings by author; joint authors or multiple authors are usually cross-referenced. Classification catalogues list the entire holdings usually as they appear on the shelves in the library. The order is determined by the classification system used.

If the library uses a manual indexing system, the information will be held on postcard-sized records stored in a series of boxes that are readily accessible. If a computer system is in place, the information will be stored on a database that can be searched by subject, author or classification code. Although the same system is used for books, journals and audio-visual stock, it is usual to keep the catalogues separate or at least to indicate the medium separately so as to assist in retrieval.

Printed indexes, abstracts and bibliographies

It has already been acknowledged that any one library can hold only a small selection of the total literature available at any time. However, by use of indexes, abstracts and bibliographies a user can identify relevant material on an international basis that can then be sought via inter-library loan or from other sources.

Printed indexes

As the name suggests, printed indexes list all material that has been published in a preselected group of journals. Both author(s) and subject heading(s) are used to index the articles. Indexes, depending on the specific publication, are produced monthly, bimonthly or quarterly, and are cumulated annually. A wide selection of indexes are available, and some, such as *Index Medicus*, list articles from almost 4000 journals. For a particular area of interest it is worth seeking advice from a librarian as to the index that will comprehensively cover the journals most likely to yield articles of relevance. Although, if time permits, users can consult more than one index, it is worth bearing in mind that there are often large areas of overlap between the various indexes.

The amount of information recorded in the index about a particular article is limited and essentially similar to that available within a standard reference, that is, name of author(s), date of publication, title of article, name of journal, volume and issue numbers, and page numbers of article. The paucity of information can be problematic, for often what seems on the basis of the title to be a valuable reference turns out to be only of peripheral or no value.

Abstracts

Abstracting journals have a significant advantage over indexes in that they provide, in addition to the reference-type information, an abstract of the article. This will enable readers to assess more accurately the potential value of a piece of work without having to access it directly. The quality of the abstract provided can, however, vary considerably from a basic outline to a detailed summary of the entire article. A wide selection of abstracts are available that can be of value to the health professional. They include *Hospital Abstracts*, *Health Service*

Abstracts, *Social Service Abstracts*, *Quality Assurance Abstracts* and *Excerpta Medica*.

Bibliographies

Bibliographies are often produced by organizations or libraries on predetermined subjects. They are essentially a reference list of books, periodical articles, reports and circulars on specific topics. In many cases these bibliographies will include limited circulation reports: for example the Scottish Health Service Centre Library regularly publishes such specialist bibliographies.

Citation indexes

Indexes, abstracts and bibliographies simply list all the material published irrespective of its quality. Citation indexes list only those articles that have been cited by other authors in their work. Such indexes record the number of times a particular article has been cited, listing in which publication it was referenced, the volume, issue and page numbers, and by whom it was cited. Entries are listed by author.

By examining the number of times a particular article has been cited it is possible to speculate about the quality of the work and/or identify topics that are of current interest to a profession. Authors of articles can also use a citation index as a means of identifying potential colleagues with a similar interest. For example, authors can examine who has cited their work, contact them, and thus extend their professional network.

MANUAL OR COMPUTER SEARCHING

Until relatively recently most libraries used manual systems. With the advent of cheap, powerful and reliable computer technology many libraries have computerized their subject index, author and classification catalogues and hold the information on a database. A database can simply be thought of as an electronic card index that can store and retrieve information in an extremely efficient and flexible manner. Not only will a database hold all the usual information expected of the index or catalogue, but also it can record whether the book is in stock, out on loan, or reserved for a subscriber. Users can search the catalogue for material on a particular subject or subjects, print a reference list of those found, and even request that those on loan be reserved on their return to the library.

Similarly, indexes, abstracts and bibliographies are now available via computer. These can be accessed either by telephoning a central computer (on-line systems) or by using CD-ROM technology on a local personal computer. Both on-line and CD-ROM systems are more expensive than their manual counterparts. Libraries have to take out a subscription to use the database, must possess the appropriate technology, and in the case of on-line services must pay telephone rental and connect charges. Because of the additional charges associated with on-line facilities, most libraries will not allow users access to such systems themselves but will perform a search for users. CD-ROM systems are usually accessible to most users since there are no additional costs.

Computer systems have the distinct advantage that they can save a tremendous amount of time, are far more flexible, can produce printed lists of references on request, and are usually more up to date than their manual counterparts. However, CD-ROM and on-line systems do have the disadvantages of high initial cost and the need for users to be computer literate and to have keyboard skills and a knowledge of the appropriate commands to conduct the search.

CONDUCTING A SEARCH

Literature searching, with a little thought and good planning, can be relatively easy. The process does, however, have to be systematic, comprehensive and unhurried if optimum results are to be obtained. When conducting a literature search it is necessary to think around the subject. Keywords and their synonyms need to be generated that adequately describe the topic to be searched for.

Although a manual search can be conducted, it is well worth while trying to obtain access to a library that has computer search facilities. This will save time and give the option of using search strategies that include more than one subject heading at one time. To search using more than one keyword at a time, 'logical operators', most commonly AND and OR, are used. By use of these logical operators a search for a combination of subjects simultaneously can be undertaken. Example 12 provides an illustrative example of a CD-ROM-based literature search.

Example 12

Illustrative example of CD-ROM-based literature search

Command	References
FIND Outcome	1342
FIND Psychiatric	111034
FIND Outcome AND Psychiatric	37

The more specific the search criteria the fewer references that are found. Too many references are clearly unmanageable and many will be of only marginal interest. Too few and it is likely that the search has missed some valuable material. The use of computer technology does not guarantee that references found are exactly relevant to the writer's needs. Only once an article is read can a reader be sure of its value.

CONCLUSIONS

Knowing what literature is available, where to look for it and how to find it are perhaps the fundamental steps in ensuring that any paper a writer plans to write will be well researched. Only by considering previous authors' publications on a subject can a writer know if they have a unique contribution to make. Although there are many sources of literature and the volume of material is immense, a systematic and comprehensive literature search, using either manual or computer techniques, can provide the budding writer with a manageable and specific pool of articles to draw upon. Literature searching is a key skill required by anyone wishing to produce scholarly work.

Chapter 7
Literature Review

Most good professional writing is based upon a detailed and rigorous evaluation of previously published literature. In Chapter 6 the knowledge, process and skills required to identify and gather literature were reviewed. In this chapter these are extended to include a detailed knowledge of the structure of professional writing and the complementary skills of literature criticism and synthesis which are an essential part of any author's toolkit.

The skills of criticism and synthesis are not just essential to the production of a new scholarly piece of work but also enable writers to recognize when a previously published piece of work is of a high standard. To enable writers to assess systematically the strengths and weaknesses of any paper, a comprehensive and ordered approach is required. If such an approach is not followed, there is a real danger that a literature review will be inconsistent, possibly biased and probably based on subjective assessment.

Evaluating literature and producing a comprehensive, objective and well argued review requires a high degree of concentration, an ordered mind and some peace and quiet. When reading material for pleasure it does not matter too much if there is an interruption by the telephone or a colleague wanting assistance. For those attempting to review material critically, such an interruption can result in a break in concentration and wasted time, and may necessitate rereading the paper. Hence it is advisable to find a spot where interruptions should not occur, where plenty of space to work is available and which, over time, can be associated with doing scholarly work. An adequate supply of paper, pencils and highlighting pens should be at hand. With these supplies and of course the paper(s) intended for review, the scene is set to commence a structured systematic critique.

CRITIQUING PUBLICATIONS

When writing a professional paper, writers often refer to a wide variety of sources. Published articles, books, reports and theses may all be consulted by an author in an attempt to identify the current knowledge base relating to the topic being written about. Whilst there are differences in the structure and layout of the various published forms, there is, fortunately, a high degree of similarity which enables the experienced or even novice author to review literature in a relatively standard, efficient and effective way. For the purpose of this chapter the structure of a research paper is used as an illustrative example. It is important to note that not all the subsections present in a research report will appear in other scholarly work.

By having a knowledge of the structure and format followed in most published work, writers can readily scan material so as to be able to identify quickly and easily the relative value of papers. This should allow a writer to judge whether the investment of time in detailed reading is warranted.

Scanning an article is not a haphazard process and needs to be systematic and thorough if material is to be discarded confidently without detailed reading. With practice it is possible to examine a full page at a time and scan from left to right while simultaneously moving from top to bottom of the page. The start of each paragraph should always be examined for words or phrases that might give clues to the content. Particular attention must be paid to all headings, bold, under-lined, enlarged or in italics, and any illustrations, graphs or tables must be closely examined. In the case of longer pieces of work such as books, theses or lengthy reports, the contents list and the index should always be used as a means of appraising the potential worth of the document. The reader should dip into the most promising sections and scan the contents as previously described. Any sections, paragraphs or sentences that signal recommendation or conclusions should be read in full and can be identified by phrases that include words such as 'in conclusion', 'therefore', 'it is recommended', 'hence', and 'it is suggested'.

Most scholarly articles follow a relatively consistent format. The for-mat is usually dictated by the journal's guide to contributors which can be found at least annually in many professional publications. This guide should assist in identifying those sections of a published paper that are most likely to yield valuable information. It should also clarify whether the author was under any specific restriction on the content, for example 'keep references to less than five and tables or figures to no more than two'. If such restrictions exist, they can prevent an author from including a comprehensive literature review and from illustrating the paper with a selection of illustrations and graphs.

Title

When considering the title of a publication, it is important to assess whether it clearly indicates the content and preferably the methodology used. The title should be succinct and able to attract any reader with an interest in the subject and entice them to read on. Cryptic or irrelevant titles that contain significant and important material may be unintentionally or prematurely discounted by a potential reader who simply scans the title. Conversely, the use of a title that contains vague and poorly defined terms in a non-standard way can result in an interested potential reader spending considerable time trying to track down and access the work only to find that the paper has no relevance to the topic under study.

Author(s)

By reviewing the author's credentials additional information may be gleaned. For example, assessing the current job title of the individual, their professional qualifications and any academic credentials should allow the reader to assess the potential relevance of his or her past experience and hence the likelihood of discovering a well written, scholarly piece of work. In some cases when an author has written extensively on a subject it may even be worthwhile considering the role of that individual when they are not the first author. Multiple authorship of papers usually indicates that there has been a need for specialist input at various points, which can add significantly to the quality of the publication. However, this is not always the case and sometimes additional authors are simply added as a means of acknowledging the assistance those individuals have given, for example in collecting data or reviewing early drafts of the paper.

Abstract

The abstract of any paper should be seen as the shop window and therefore should always be read when attempting to evaluate the paper's worth. A well constructed abstract should present in approximately 100 to 500 words an overview of the major points of the paper including background, issues addressed, method employed, major findings and any conclusions or recommendations. Some journals also now request that the author provide a number of keywords which any interested party might use to search for the work. These are usually included at the end of the abstract in bold type and can be an excellent guide to the potential reader as to whether the paper addresses the topic of interest.

Introduction

The introduction of any paper should set the scene, clearly identifying the problem that is being addressed and providing a rationale for the work. Any difficulties encountered or limitations to the extent of the work may also be addressed within this section. If an abstract is not available, the introduction should be read carefully since it should be possible to assess the paper's applicability to the topic under review.

Literature review

As previously mentioned, journals often place strict limits on the length and format of any literature review. It is therefore important to assess, by reading the guide to contributors, whether what may appear superficial and incomplete is in fact a result of the journal's house style and not caused by a lack of understanding of the subject on the author's part.

In general, in the case of books, dissertations and research reports, an author should provide a complete and detailed review of the literature. In particular both the conceptual framework(s) underpinning any previous work as well as the associated findings should be adequately compared and contrasted. The structure of the review should, as a rule, move from the general topic area to the specific issues being considered. A literature review should always consider the topic from all perspectives and should not simply present evidence to support the author's viewpoint. If contrasting views do not exist, it needs to be pointed out by the author that, despite searching for such views, none has been found.

Papers that cite work that is old may indicate that the work was conducted some time ago, that the author is unfamiliar with current literature, or that there has been a delay in the publication process. Most scholarly journals should state clearly when the paper was accepted for publication, and this date should be used to assess whether the literature presented can be considered current.

Unfortunately, some papers are published that provide an incomplete review of the literature. To a reader who is fully familiar with a subject the omission of seminal work in the field can be glaringly obvious. Great care must be taken when assessing such an article since it could suggest that the work has been based on an incomplete review of the literature. In such cases the conclusions reached may be only partially correct or, in the worst cases, totally incorrect. Although unlikely, it may be that the omission by the author was deliberate and a consequence of an inability to see a way of incorporating such seminal work meaningfully into the review.

The hypothesis

When reviewing a study that uses an experimental methodology, the author should disclose and clearly state the hypothesis which is to be tested by the study. In some cases, in addition to the main hypothesis there may be further linked sub-hypotheses. In all cases the hypothesis must be phrased in a manner that is capable of being tested and stated in terms that are totally unambiguous. It is important to note that a great deal of research does not use experimental designs and therefore will not have a hypothesis. In such cases, however, a research question(s) should be clearly stated.

Operational definitions

When reviewing specialized literature it is important to recognize that everyday terms can have very specific and often unique meaning. It is therefore essential that if terms are used that are in any way open to interpretation, appropriate operational definitions are stated by the author. Without such definitions, readers and even the subjects of the paper may use their own, personal definition of the terms being used, and this may, in the very worst of cases, invalidate findings. For example, the word 'treatment' may mean a physical intervention such as applying a bandage, or a psychological intervention such as reflecting back the feeling content of a conversation. Obviously, if there is no clear definition of the term 'treatment', this introduces unacceptable ambiguity in a paper addressing such an issue as the effectiveness of treatment outcome.

Methodology

When reviewing a paper, appropriate consideration should be given to the methodology section. If comprehensively written this should give sufficient information to enable the reader to develop a clear understanding of the approach followed, and to allow the work to be replicated if necessary. The methods section usually consists of a number of subsections that should allow the reader to put the rest of the article in context.

Subjects

To compare and contrast a previously published piece of work effectively, it is vital that the reader be fully aware of the characteristics of the individuals or situations that have been studied. A clear and detailed understanding should enable the reader to judge whether the subjects of the study under review have relevance to the issue, group or facility that is being studied and the potential for local applicability.

Sample selection

A clear statement of the mechanism used to recruit individuals or situations is required. For example, the use of a convenience sample is likely to result in findings that may have only local significance and may be biased in some way. Conversely, random selection of subjects should produce data that can be extrapolated to other settings. Whilst the sample size will be dependent on many factors, not least the design and objectives of the study, readers should give due consideration to this matter, particularly if the author intends to extrapolate the results to a wider population.

In some types of research design the exact number of subjects to be recruited will not be known at the outset, for example in the case of studies that employ a grounded theory approach. However, in such cases the author should give a clear statement on the criteria to be used to decide when 'enough' subjects have been recruited. Sample selection is a critical factor in deciding whether the results of an article are likely to have relevance in another setting, as is any subsequent information on any difficulty in recruiting subjects. Such difficulties may result in the study being based on a self-selected and possibly biased group which may be atypical of the intended subjects of the study.

Data collection

Questionnaires, interviews, documentary analysis, focus groups, observation or measurement are all approaches that can be used in the process of data collection. Some approaches are more appropriate to a particular study design than others, and it is within this context that the reader must consider the relevance of the data collection methods. The method selected should be compatible with the underlying theoretical framework and the aims of the study.

If instruments such as questionnaires are being used, the author should present evidence that sufficient pilot study work has been undertaken and that the validity and reliability of the measures are sufficiently robust for the particular setting and subjects. Failure to pilot and to consider the validity and reliability of the measurement processes and tools can result in data that are questionable. Sadly, it is common to read in the literature that researchers have used previously tried and tested questionnaires with established validity and reliability but have assumed, quite wrongly, that these measures are applicable in a totally different setting or with a different subject group.

Data analysis

Data analysis is not something that is decided on once the data have been collected. A well written and designed study should demonstrate that sufficient forethought and planning have gone into devising the analysis well before data are collected. Some researchers may even go as far as generating dummy data to test out the procedures as part of pilot work. If dummy data are used, a description of how they were generated or obtained should be presented.

Ethical considerations

The rights of subjects are of prime importance. Whether the researcher is using patients, people doing their weekly shopping, or students, the ethical implications of the study should be addressed. Although procedures for gaining ethical approval to conduct any study involving human subjects will differ from place to place, evidence should be presented to indicate that ethical approval was sought and obtained. The approval of a research and ethics committee, if such is properly constituted, can also give the reader additional confidence that the study has at least met some minimum standards and is not likely to contain major methodological flaws.

Results or findings

Results, sometimes referred to as findings, should be presented in a clear, concise, accurate and logical manner. The reader should always bear in mind the original aims of the paper and question whether or not the research results address these in sufficient detail to enable a conclusive statement to be made. If statistical tests are used, the reader should check that these are appropriate to the data and the design of the study. If graphs, tables and diagrams are used to present the data, it is important that they be sufficiently and accurately labelled and supported by explanations within the text to allow the reader to interpret correctly the significance of the information being presented.

The results section can stand alone but some authors integrate this with the discussion. In a research paper or thesis the results section should simply present the data obtained with subsequent sections building upon the evidence discovered. A complete detailed examination and understanding of the results is necessary if a critical appraisal of the remaining parts of the paper is to be made.

Discussion

The purpose of the discussion is to explore and interpret the results obtained in the study. It also gives the author the opportunity to compare and contrast the findings of the study with any other relevant previously reported or published material. The discussion should identify any weaknesses in the design and preferably propose how these could be avoided if the study were to be repeated. A discussion should be a full, frank, balanced and objective discourse on the issues being investigated and the results obtained.

Conclusions

The conclusions section of any report is of great significance to any reader who is trying to assess the worth and relevance of a paper. Many readers may, in the absence of an abstract or where the abstract is brief, turn to the conclusions section to judge whether time should be invested in detailed reading of the paper. Conclusions should be clearly presented and supported by the results and subsequent discussion, and should provide a balanced ending to the report by acknowledging strengths, weaknesses and any flaws in the design, conduct or outcome of the study.

Recommendations

Recommendations should be clear, concise and based upon the evidence presented in the paper. The recommendations may relate to a change in practice or more commonly should advocate the need for further studies to be conducted. Care must be taken to ensure that the writer has not advocated action that is not supported by the evidence presented.

Reference list

Any scholarly work should build on previous literature. The reference list should include, usually, up to date material. On some occasions older work will be cited but this should be material that is seminal or central to the development of the writer's arguments. References should be set out in keeping with the requirements of the journal in which the article is published and should always give sufficient information to enable an interested reader to get a copy.

Appendices

It is unusual to see appendices published as part of articles that appear in journals. They are more common in books, research reports and theses. Appendices should contain material that gives the reader an opportunity to examine in greater depth an issue covered in the main paper, for example a specimen copy of a research instrument such as a questionnaire. Appendices can be a particularly rich source of information for anyone wishing to replicate previous work.

RECORDING A CRITICAL EVALUATION

Having spent considerable time evaluating the worth and relevance of an article it is essential that all relevant information obtained be stored in a systematic manner that should enable the later recall and use of the material and perhaps even allow the reader to integrate other material at a later date.

One approach is to write this information in a standard format on a small card that can be stored alphabetically by author or subject covered. With the ready availability of information technology an electronic solution is to use a relational database. This has the advantage over a manual card system that material can be searched by any of a number of ways that may yield the result desired: by author, date, title, journal or keywords.

Irrespective of whether a manual or electronic solution is used to store the evaluation, it is essential that a certain minimum amount of data be noted down accurately. For example, in the case of books, the data should include the author(s), date of publication, title, editor(s), edition, place of publication and publisher. In the case of journal articles it is essential that the journal title, volume and part numbers and the pages of the article be accurately recorded. Irrespective of source it will be necessary to record the critical review of the content and perhaps how the work relates to other material in the field of study. Example 13 gives a suggested layout for the storing of reference material. If a computer database is used, it is also worth while noting some keywords that can be of assistance when recalling groups of articles characterized by the particular keyword, for example NHS reforms or childhood illnesses. Whilst it can be useful to develop original keyword categories, readers may wish to use already established categories such as those used by commercially available indexing services, for example *Index Medicus.*

Example 13   _____

Format for recording essential reference information

Author(s):	Year of publication:
Title:	

Journal:

Volume:	Part No:	Pages:	Place of publication:
Publisher:			Editor(s):

Keywords:
Synopsis of paper:

_____

WRITING A LITERATURE REVIEW

The writing and structuring of a literature review is dependent upon the ability to critique individual articles. More importantly it is the integration of the individual critiques that provides the aspiring writer with the greatest challenge.

A well written literature review does not consist of a simple serial list of individual critiques. It should be a synthesis that distils the essence of the work reviewed. It should provide the reader with a balanced picture of the strengths, weaknesses and gaps in the knowledge base being considered. The review must be presented in an objective manner which supports any criticisms with appropriate evidence. Both material that endorses and refutes the author's position should be presented and effectively discussed. A literature review should provide a basis upon which a clear decision can be made as to the need for further work in the field of study. It is therefore of central importance and should be seen as the foundation of scholarly writing.

THE STRUCTURE OF A LITERATURE REVIEW

The previous section described the objectives of a literature review. It is important to consider the exact format that such a section should take. Researching the topic may have taken many hours, days, weeks or months of sifting through articles in preparation for writing the review. It is therefore essential that due care and attention be given to the structure if a well integrated, tightly argued and coherent paper is to be produced.

The structure of a literature review is relatively simple. First, there should be an introduction that sets the scene by describing the sources consulted and that indicates the time span covered by the critiqued papers. If time limits are set, outside of which published material was not considered, the rationale for these must be given.

Secondly, the main body of the review should contain the synthesis of previously published material which should address the theoretical frameworks used and the associated research evidence available. Whenever possible the author should paraphrase previous work although direct quotations may be used to emphasize central issues. However, quotes can interrupt the flow of the text. Furthermore, when taken out of context they may lose their significance or, worse still, be interpreted differently by the reader.

A well organized review that identifies a number of competing theoretical frameworks within the area of study should deal with these in a systematic manner. Consideration of the strengths and weaknesses and the areas of similarity and difference, of the various publications reviewed should be given, and any previous research results should be used to underpin observations or arguments being presented. Gaps or inconsistencies should be clearly identified and explored. Any article(s) seen as central to the development of arguments should be dealt with in depth.

Thirdly, the review should conclude with a summary of the findings of the critique. This final part of the review should provide the rationale for conducting further studies or for a change in practice if unequivocal evidence is discovered.

Inadequate analysis and synthesis of literature often results in a review that appears to be simply a series of disjointed paragraphs which merely echo the words of previous authors. Professional writing that enables the boundaries of knowledge to be advanced is characterized by a well structured, systematic, logical and coherent approach.

Chapter 8
Illustrations

Illustrations are any form of presentation, other than straightforward prose or mathematical formulae, used to add to the impact of the written word. They include photographs, tables, line drawings, flow charts and other illustrative forms. Some works are incomplete without illustrations, others do not need them, and in others they might be optional. The author decides whether unillustrated words are adequate, or whether additional visual material is necessary. In any event the decision to include or exclude illustrations is a conscious one. The important question is: 'Are illustrations needed to enhance the quality of the work and, if so, which one(s) will add to its readability and clarity?'.

Although the writer is often able to make decisions about the use and possible choice of illustrations, it may be worth while discussing this with a graphic artist or photographer. Because a wide range of sophisticated illustrations are produced by computer graphics technology, the writer should seriously consider discussing its use with someone with knowledge of the field. If the work is being prepared for publication, the inclusion of illustrations must be discussed with the publisher at an early stage as some place restrictions on the size, type and colour, for example. Illustration use also has financial implications which publishers wish to take into account.

In coursework and dissertations, which are not for publication, each illustration must be placed in the text close to the point at which it is first referred to. If insufficient room for it remains on the page, it should be placed on the next one. In either event, reference to the illustration might read, for example: 'Figure 1 shows the distribution of marks between respondents', or 'Figure 5 demonstrates the differences between the posture of elderly men and young men'.

If the material is being prepared for publication, the publisher's 'Guide for authors' may request that illustrations be incorporated into the text as described in the preceding paragraph. More commonly, publishers ask that they be placed at the end of the text with full instructions as to where they should appear in the work. If the illustrations are to be placed at the end of the text, they should each be placed on a different page and identified by their figure number and title. They should be numbered according to the chapter in which they appear, the first figure in Chapter 5 being labelled Figure 5.1, for example. The text will contain a clear indication of where each illustration is to be inserted by including a statement such as 'Place Fig. 1 near here please'.

Because the illustrations used in this book are *examples* of, rather than actual, tables, figures and the like, they are referred to as Example 1, Example 2, and so on.

The convention is that all illustrations apart from tables are referred to as figures.

TABLES

Tables are used to present numerical information in summary form, and like text are read from left to right. They are probably the most widely used and abused form of illustration; because of their popularity, many writers wrongly assume that little thought needs to be given to producing them. As with all forms of illustration, tables require careful thought and planning. Example 14 illustrates a number of common errors which are made in constructing tables. Although it is unusual for all errors to appear in the same table, each is relatively common.

Example 14

Common errors in tables

Distribution of patients' ages

Age		Numbers	% In Each Group
0–20 yrs	(1)	192	22.994%
21–40 yrs		225	26.946%
41–60 yrs		109 (3)	13.05%
61–80 yrs		184	22%
81 + yrs	(2)	125	14.97%

NOTE
(1) The youngest patient was aged 8 yrs and 4 months on the day of the survey.
(2) The oldest patient was aged 102 yrs and six months on the day of the survey.
(3) Includes one patient on holiday on the day of the survey.

The deliberate errors in the table shown in Example 14 are as follows.

Heading. The table heading is not sufficiently descriptive of the contents of the table. A more appropriate title would be 'Distribution of patients by age on 1 January 1993: District General Hospital'. Each table must be numbered according to the chapter in which it appears. Thus the first table in Chapter 4 would be numbered 4.1. Table numbering permits more accurate cross reference in the text and, if the work is to be published, placement of the complete table as near to its text reference as possible avoids having to turn from one page to another.

First column. The use of abbreviations within a table is strongly discouraged when, as in this case, there is ample room for the items to be written out in full. If an abbreviation is used, the term must be written in full followed by the abbreviation in parentheses on the first occasion of use, for example 'years (yrs)' and the abbreviation used thereafter. As with the table, each column requires a full and descriptive heading. 'Age' is inadequate and is improved upon in the next example.

Second column. It is customary to indicate, where appropriate, the total number of items that will appear in a column. This should have been done as '(Total = 835)'.

Third column. The numbers in this and other columns must be presented consistently and in correct alignment so as to minimize possible confusion. Thus each item is calculated to the same number of places after the decimal point. Also, the decimal point of each entry needs to be aligned exactly with all others in that column. Finally, there is no need to present the per cent sign (%) in relation to each entry; the % sign in the column heading will suffice.

Example 15 _____

Correction of common errors in tables

Distribution of patients by age on 1 January 1993:
District General Hospital

Age on 1 Jan 1993 (years)	Numbers of patients (Total=835)	% of total patients in each age group (1)
0–20 (2)	192	23
21–40	225	27
41–60	109 (3)	13
61–80	184	22
80 + (4)	125	15
Totals	835	100

Notes
(1) Figures in this column have been 'rounded up' to the nearest whole number.
(2) The youngest patient was aged 8 years and 4 months on the day of the survey.
(3) Includes one patient on holiday on the day of the survey.
(4) The oldest patient was 102 years and 6 months on the day of the survey.

Space. A common error is to concentrate too much material into the space occupied by a table. The first example contains the same volume of material as does the second. However, the space allocated to the second is substantially greater. If the information is too much to place into one table in a visually attractive way, additional tables should be used.

Table footnote. When it is desirable to enliven facts with additional information but not to increase the size of the table with more columns, a table footnote may be used. The table footnote references (asterisks, daggers and the like or letters or numbers) are used to connect the table footnote with the item in the table. When letters or numbers are used, their sequence should read from left to right as the table is read, and not from top to the bottom of a column.

Totals. Below each column containing percentage or other values, a total of the values in the column is required.

Example 15 corrects the deliberate errors made in Example 14.

TYPES OF FIGURES

Pie chart

The pie chart is most often used to show proportional distributions such as the percentage distribution of patients in various age groups. The tools required to construct a pie chart are: a pair of compasses or some other means of drawing a perfect circle, a protractor for dividing the circle into its predetermined parts, paper and a pencil. Alternatively, a computer graphics package might be used.

In constructing the pie chart the size of each of its sections is calculated as follows. Each $1\% = 3.6°$ (3.6 being 1% of the 360° circumference of the circle). Thus 192 (23%) of the patients are aged between 0 and 20 years, therefore 3.6×23 of the chart (83°) relates to patients in that age group.

The pie chart is only used when there is a smaller rather than a larger number of items to be included. If the number of items is in excess of ten, for example, the large number of relatively small parts will be difficult to distinguish from each other. Similarly, as parts of the pie become smaller and represent tiny percentages, 1% for example, it becomes very difficult to indicate to the reader the value of such parts.

The contents of the pie chart can be entered either within the pie chart, as in Example 16, or outside it with a line from the item to the appropriate part of the chart. Alternatively, a colour or some other form of coding such as lines or dots can be used within the chart, and an appropriate key and caption placed immediately below or to the side of the chart.

Example 16

Pie chart

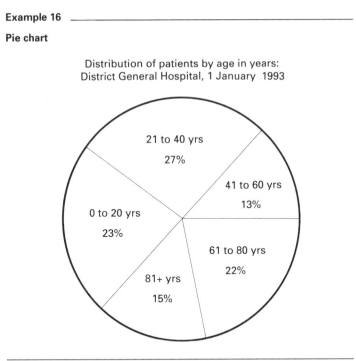

Distribution of patients by age in years:
District General Hospital, 1 January 1993

21 to 40 yrs
27%

41 to 60 yrs
13%

0 to 20 yrs
23%

61 to 80 yrs
22%

81+ yrs
15%

Contour plot

Contour plots are used to demonstrate the changes in surface area that have occurred over time. For example, the effect of treatment on the granulation of a decubitus ulcer at various time intervals can be recorded as in Example 17. This form of illustration would provide an objective and relatively accurate record of the rate of healing.

Line drawing

Line drawings are often used to illustrate the type of material that would otherwise be conveyed by photographs. Although they never have the quality of photographs, they have the advantage of not requiring the agreement of their human 'subjects' or their permission to publish. In some instances a line drawing may be the best way of illustrating an idea or event. For example, it is probably the best means of demonstrating anatomical and physiological subjects such as the production of urine by the kidneys, the transfer of urine to the urinary bladder and the expulsion of urine via the urethra.

As the construction of a good quality line drawing is outside the skill of all but the most artistic of writers, it is more usual to employ an artist for the purpose. Example 18 shows typical finished artwork of such a

Example 17

Contour plot

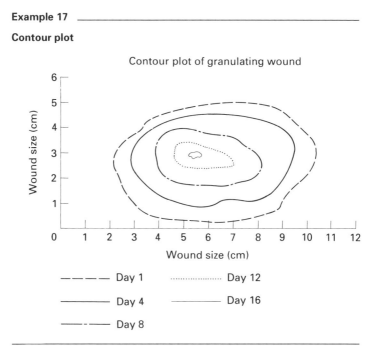

Contour plot of granulating wound

————— Day 1   ·············· Day 12

————— Day 4   ——— Day 16

—·—·— Day 8

Example 18

Line drawing

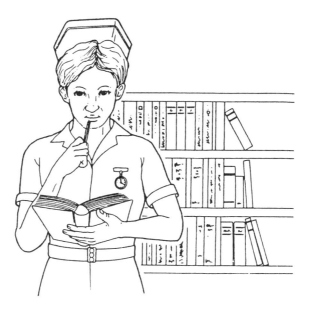

commissioned drawing which carried the request: 'Draw a 30-year-old female nurse looking at a book in a library'.

Line drawings required for a book are not commissioned until the author has discussed them with the publisher or editor, who may prefer to have the final artwork done in house by the publisher. The reasons for this range from technical to aesthetic, and all that may be needed from the author is clearly labelled rough pencil drawings.

Flow chart

Many writers use flow charts to convey to readers the relationship and sequence of individual ideas that form part of a larger concept. Flow charts have a definite beginning and end point, each being clearly defined to enable readers to understand how the sequence of events starts and ends. Correct flow-chart layout is important if clarity of presentation and information flow are to be ensured. The best and most easily understood flow charts read from top to bottom, with feedback loops going in the reverse direction. In Example 19, activities are included in rectangular boxes and decision points are indicated by diamond shapes.

Common errors seen in the production of flow charts include the omission of decision points and of arrows to guide the reader through the chart, and the crossover of feedback paths over earlier sections of the chart.

Line graph

Line graphs are particularly useful for displaying changes over time. It is necessary to ensure that the time intervals along the horizontal axis are equal. A common error in line graph use is the omission of any discontinuities in the scale. That is, if the first scale point is 55, as is the case in Example 20, then the discontinuity between '0' and '60' must be shown as indicated in the example.

Geographic mapping

This type of illustration is most useful when a writer wishes to indicate the distribution of an item relative to a geographic area of an entire country, region or even more local area.

Geographic mapping can easily be produced by hand but with new technology it is possible to translate information directly from data files into this format by means of a suitable software package.

Example 21 shows the population density of people aged 65 years or more in the geographical subdivisions of a hospital catchment area.

Example 19

Flow chart

Organization, delivery and evaluation of care

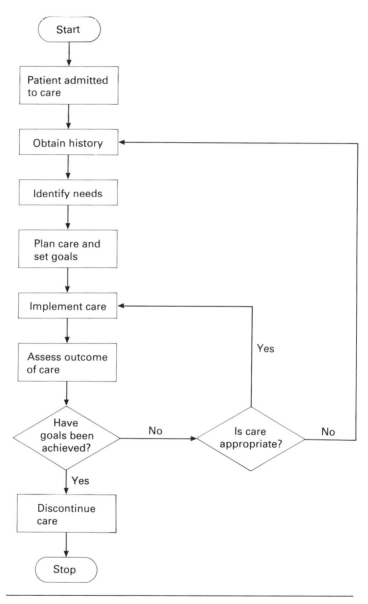

Example 20

Line graph

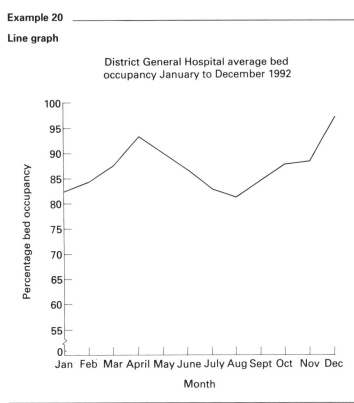

District General Hospital average bed occupancy January to December 1992

Sociograms

Sociograms are useful means of describing the frequency with which individuals interact with each other. Such a description does not require an illustration if a small number of participants are involved in the interaction, for example two. However, the difficulties of presenting and understanding an unillustrated description of interaction frequency among ten or more participants are easy to imagine.

In constructing a sociogram, decisions must be made regarding the individuals to whom it will relate and the information it will contain. In Example 22 the one-to-one interactions between a teacher and students have been recorded, solid lines indicating those initiated by the teacher and broken lines representing student-initiated interactions. The percentage figure in each of the peripheral circles represents the amount of one-to-one interaction time involving each individual student.

The sociogram is a highly specialized form of presentation which allows easy identification of individuals who rarely or never interact (*isolates*) and those who frequently interact (*stars*).

When the number of people to be included in a sociometric illustration is large, the use of several sociograms might be preferable to

Example 21 _____

Geographic map

Distribution of elderly population (65 years+)
in catchment area of District General Hospital

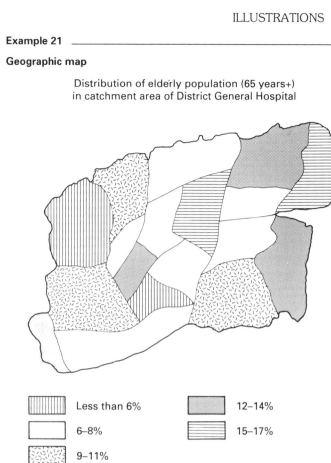

▥ Less than 6%		▨ 12–14%	
☐ 6–8%		☰ 15–17%	
▦ 9–11%			

placing all the information in a single illustration. There is no hard and fast rule regarding the acceptable complexity of a sociogram; trial and error should precede the final decision.

Bar graph

The bar graph also presents numerical data in pictorial form. It can either be horizontal or vertical; Example 23 is of the former type.

The individual bars in the graph each represent one part of the data. They are drawn to scale and are separate from each other. Each part of the graph is labelled, with the item to which the bar refers being placed close to the base of the bar. The axis relating to measurement (the horizontal axis in this instance) is drawn to scale.

Organizational chart

The organizational chart (see Example 24) presents the relationship between individuals, positions or various parts of an organization. This

Example 22

Sociogram

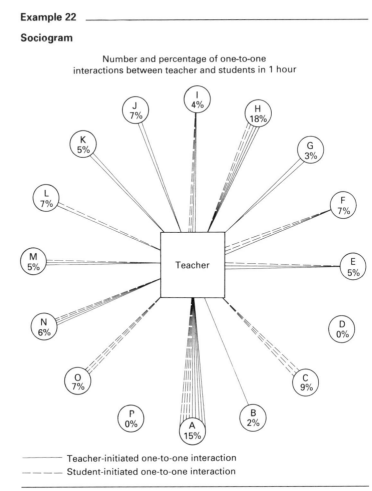

Number and percentage of one-to-one
interactions between teacher and students in 1 hour

——————— Teacher-initiated one-to-one interaction

– – – – – Student-initiated one-to-one interaction

is a further example of the use of a technique to present information which would be difficult to understand in prose form. Simplicity of presentation is an essential feature of the organizational chart. Material which is too complex for a single chart is placed on two or more separate charts.

Blueprint

Blueprints are used to indicate the size, general structure, position and spatial relationships of areas such as rooms, houses or wards. Example 25 shows a blueprint of a ward, not drawn to scale, indicating the major parts.

The content of this form of illustration depends on what is to be drawn to the attention of the reader; examples include hard/soft floor coverings, forms of wall coverings, free access and locked areas, and

Example 23

Bar graph

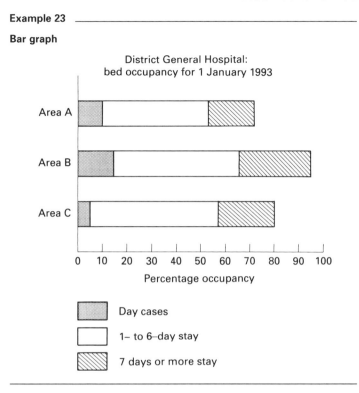

District General Hospital:
bed occupancy for 1 January 1993

Example 24

Organizational chart

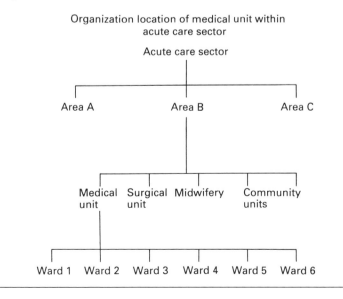

Organization location of medical unit within
acute care sector

distances between key areas in the ward. If, as is the case in Example 25, the intention is only to indicate the relative position of each of the rooms in the ward, it is not necessary to include the location of individual beds, wash-hand basins, windows and so on.

Example 25

Blueprint

Blueprint of ward (not to scale)

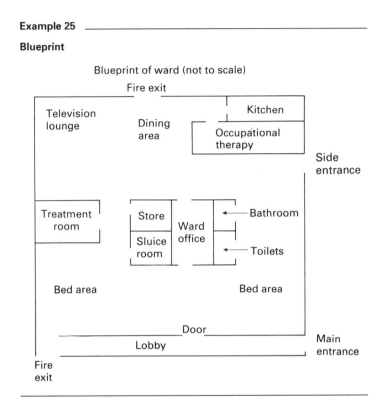

Photographs

Because photographs can be expensive to include in a work, many publishers wish them to be kept to a minimum or not included. When they are accepted, they invariably have to be black and white. Colour, being much more expensive to publish, is reserved for subjects such as dermatology which require it.

High-quality black-and-white photographs in the size range 152 mm × 101 mm to 254 mm × 204 mm (6 in × 4 in to 10 in × 8 in) should be submitted unmounted and uncut. Any instructions, for example the figure number, must be written on a sticky label before it is stuck to the back of the photograph. Paperclips or staples must never be used to attach material as they will leave marks which appear on reproduction. If the photograph has to be cut or cropped to a smaller size, this is left to the publisher, who uses either a mark on the back in crayon to indicate the material to be used or marks a photocopy. If there could be any doubt to the publisher or printer as to which is the top edge, this should also be indicated in crayon on the back. It is very important to ensure that any marks made on the rear of one photograph do not transfer on to the good side of any adjacent photographs. Thus the use of ballpoint pen to label photographs is unadvisable.

Photographs can often be used to describe something which is virtually impossible to capture in words – human feelings or a landscape for example – and can add an obvious 'human touch' to a paper. As with other illustrations, photographs should only be included if they add to the quality of the work.

Packaging used to send photographs to the publisher should be such that no damage can be done to the contents. When necessary, particularly if human subjects are used in the photography, formal written permission to publish the photograph may be necessary from the person or persons shown. Alternatively, the publisher may be instructed to use a masking technique to hide the identity of subjects.

USE OF ILLUSTRATIONS

When deciding whether illustrations are necessary and, if so, which ones to use, the following points should be considered in order to optimize impact. These apply equally to articles, books or other forms of writing such as coursework, exams and research reports.

The writer should obtain and study any constraints imposed by examiners, publishers, degree-awarding bodies and the like. If instructions do not refer to the use of illustrations or do not answer specific questions, the appropriate individual should be contacted regarding this point. It can be disheartening to find that time or money has been wasted on photographic illustrations only to discover that they cannot be included in submitted work.

If illustrations can be used, it is important to ask whether or not they should be used. Clearly, this question cannot be properly answered unless an author is fully aware of the purpose, advantages and variety of different types of illustration. If the material can be presented in the form of well written prose, then illustrations may detract from the work. When words alone are inadequate for the purpose, or where illustrations will add to the visual impact of a presentation, then drawings, photographs, tables and the like should be used.

The purpose of the illustration will determine the type that is used. For example, the physical features associated with the ageing process may be best conveyed with a photograph or a good line drawing. Alternatively, a table may best describe numerical information. If the most appropriate type of illustration is unclear, or more than one approach is possible, then experimentation with a number of types and discussion with colleagues or the publisher may make the choice easier.

If illustrations are used, they should be as 'independent' of the text as possible in that they have a well chosen title and require minimal explanation in the text. The amount of discussion which an illustration requires in the text must be considered carefully and never left to chance. If tables are used to summarize numerical information, the writer needs to decide how much or how little of the tabular information should be repeated in the text or as an appendix.

Illustrations should be kept as simple as possible. Long and complex tables or figures defeat the whole purpose of their use. Readers dislike complex and over-full illustrations. Ideally they should be short, sharp and to the point, and have an accurate descriptive title.

The number of illustrations used must be balanced against the total length of the text, too many being as much of a problem as too few. Although there is no hard and fast rule about their proportion in relation to text, they are probably too numerous if they exceed more than one-third of the total text length.

References to figures and tables in the text must *not* read 'In the following table', 'Table 1.5 below', 'Table 1.4 above', or 'See Table 1.5 which is presented below'. The reader is simply requested to 'See Table 1.5' or informed that 'Table 1.5 summarizes the findings . . .'. Avoiding use of terms such as 'above', 'below' and 'following' is necessary because the publisher will instruct the printer to place the illustrations as near as possible to their mention in the text, and prefers not to be constrained by the author specifying the exact location.

It must be remembered that mistakes may be made in the use of illustrations, and that these may be made by the author, the typist, the artist, the typesetter or the publisher. As with the text in general, all illustrations must be checked and rechecked.

Chapter 9
Examinations and Coursework

Although different, exams and coursework have some similarities in that both are submitted in order to pass some form of academic test, their prime purpose being to enable the writer to obtain a certificate, diploma or degree or some other academic or professional award. Despite separate discussion of both subjects in this chapter, there is considerable overlap. Also, the requirements of different institutions and of the teaching staff in them will vary. This chapter therefore offers general guidelines which might be used in addition to the more specific ones produced by the institution and/or staff for which the work is being prepared.

EXAMINATIONS

This discussion is confined to essay-type exams which are more dependent on the use of writing skills than, for example, multiple-choice objective tests. Such exams usually offer a choice of questions and allow candidates access to past papers for study purposes prior to the exam.

Past papers

Assuming that no significant change in the general format and content of the examination has taken place, it is advisable to study exam papers set during the last five years. This will help to 'get a feel' of past papers and increase familiarity with the way in which the questions are set and with the exam structure. Although in many instances teaching staff give students the opportunity to answer past papers, as part of class tests for example, additional experience in personal time can be profitable.

Most teachers are willing to mark and discuss answers to past papers which have been written by students as part of private study. Feedback from teaching staff, no matter how brief, is valuable.

Examination structure

It is usual for teaching staff to give prior notice of the structure of exams in terms of the number of questions in the paper, the number to be answered, and the general area to be covered by each of the paper's sections. It is useful to establish if possible whether or not there is to be a compulsory distribution of questions. For example, examinees might have to answer five questions in a 3-hour period, including at least one from section A, one from section B, and one from section C.

Exam preparation

Students have a personal responsibility to study, practise and know examination subjects well. Any reservations or confusion about the subject must be identified as soon as possible and discussed with staff before the exam. Thorough knowledge and experience of the subject matter do *not* guarantee the ability to write a satisfactory answer under examination conditions. Although such knowledge and experience are necessary prerequisites, it is also important to have considerable experience in answering questions, under examination conditions, prior to the actual exam.

Initially, private examination practice might be with the assistance of textbooks or course notes, or by extending the time limit. As more skill develops, the books and notes should no longer be used and the time allocated for the answers should be reduced to that available in the actual exam. Whenever possible, this type of practice work should be shown to and discussed with teaching staff or a personal tutor.

The examination

The candidate should enter the exam room with a watch and all other required materials. *Every* word of the exam paper, including intro-ductory material, instructions and all questions, must be read carefully. Every item on the exam paper must be re-read. Preliminary decisions must be made about which questions are to be answered and in which order. If the questions can be answered in any order, it may be best to start with the question that inspires most confidence.

As with other forms of writing, some thought must be given to the structure of the answer before focusing on the detail of content. It is usually permissible to do 'rough work' within the answer book. In most instances such work has to be deleted by drawing lines through it before the end of the exam. Thus, the rough work will not be regarded by the examiner as part of the answer. In addition to outlining the content, planning for the structure of the answer can be done in the form of rough work.

Ensure that enough time is left at the end of the exam for checking and rechecking all written material, particularly numerical values and calculations. Although major changes cannot be made, minor changes and corrections that may add to the quality of the answer can often be incorporated.

General hints for examinations

- The question paper must be read very carefully, paying particular attention to the distribution of marks within parts of a question. If different parts of a question are allocated varying proportions of the total marks for that question, that *may* influence the length of time and written material given to that part of the question. For example, if part A of a three-part question is allocated 10%, part B 30%, and part C 60% of that question's marks and one hour is available for answering the whole question, the candidate should consider allocating each part a pro-rata proportion of the available hour, that is, 6, 18 and 36 minutes respectively. Although such a distribution of time must be flexible, it can help to have some notion of how to allocate limited time.
- The candidate should spend some time preparing an outline of content and structure for the answer. This can be flexible but should serve as a useful guide and starting point.
- It is vital that the candidate answers the question which was asked. This means reading the question carefully three times, confining the answer to the question asked, and not 'waffling' and getting off the point.
- The candidate should not necessarily avoid a question because the answer to a small part of it is not known; he or she should be willing to admit to being uncertain on that point. For example, if the candidate is attracted to a particular question but is unable to remember a specific drug dose required in the answer, he or she should feel free to answer the question and admit that the drug dose cannot be remembered. However, the examiner will expect to be told how, under 'normal' conditions, the correct drug dose can be established.
- It is important to write clearly and legibly. Although examiners take account of the fact that material has been written under examination conditions, the manner in which answers are written and presented will influence them. Obviously, no credit can be given for answers that cannot be understood.
- Headings and subheadings should be used to break up the answer. This makes for easier reading and gives the answer a clearer structure and a more professional finish.
- The candidate should consider using references in the answer but will probably not be expected to remember full details of them or to produce a perfect reference list. This is a matter that should be discussed with examiners and/or teaching staff well in advance of the exam.
- Tables and drawings, graphs and other kinds of figure can be used in the answer. These may be optional in some cases, desirable or essential in others.

● All the time available for the exam should be used. There is rarely any excuse for leaving early: any extra time can be used for checking and rechecking answers.

As with all types of writing, answering examination questions requires not only a thorough understanding of the subject matter but also investment of time in obtaining writing practice, in this case under self-imposed examination conditions. Some students feel that self-imposed practice is unnecessary because the specific content of the exam cannot be predicted. However, the purpose of such practice is not to predict content: it is to practise writing under exam conditions and to revise the subject matter. With this kind of practice, students undoubtedly enter the examination room with more confidence and better preparation and are able to concentrate more on *content* and less on structure.

COURSEWORK

Coursework increasingly forms an integral part of several types of study. In many courses students have a continuous and often heavy course-work load. In the following discussion of coursework, the reader should bear in mind that individual institutions and teachers have their own requirements. The following material is offered in addition to those specific requirements. As with the earlier material relating to exam-inations, the requirements of teaching staff and their institutions take precedence over these guidelines.

The coursework subject

It is important to read the subject of the coursework carefully. If there are any doubts as to its meaning, or if the reader's understanding of it seems to differ from that of other students, this should be discussed immedi-ately with the person who set the work. Some coursework 'questions' are set as statements for discussion. For example:

'Making a clinical assessment is an early part of the treatment process. Discuss.'

The key words in this statement are 'clinical assessment' and 'treatment process', and must feature prominently in the answer.

Marking criteria

Teachers usually, though not always, give prior notice of coursework marking criteria. In such cases the criteria indicate the maximum marks to be allocated to each part or aspect of the work. For example, marks may be allocated to such things as use of references, structure, presentation, content, grammar and writing style, clinical application and so on. Any such instructions must be retained and referred to throughout preparation of the work. They are a useful guide to planning the coursework structure and to deciding where to place the emphasis. For example if 10% of the marks are being awarded to conclusion and discussion, it is reasonable to assume that that part will constitute approximately 10% of the coursework length. Similarly, if a proportion of the marks are allocated to the appropriate use of references and/or to the inclusion of a bibliography, it is essential that this be included. It is usual for the maximum and/or minimum length of the work to be prescribed; examiners will usually be hard on those who ignore such a stipulation.

Structure

Thought must be given to the general structure of the coursework by creating a series of headings, subheadings and sub-subheadings which will constitute the framework of the answer. Although these will be modified as the work progresses, the writer should start off with a framework in mind and on paper. An estimate of how much time, in terms of words, will be allocated to each part of the answer can be made at this point.

In coursework concerning the importance of clinical assessment as part of the treatment process, an initial structure might be as described in Example 26.

Example 26 _____

Coursework structure

Introduction
Overview of treatment process, position and function of clinical
    assessment
Discussion of assessment generally
Extended discussion of *clinical* assessment
Sources of clinical data as basis of assessment
Alternative clinical assessment strategies
Description of clinical assessment strategy preferred by the writer
Detailed discussion of role of clinical assessment in treatment process
Conclusion and general discussion
References
Bibliography

Writing the coursework

Although use will inevitably be made of class notes, references provided during lectures, and the prescribed reading for the course, examiners will expect to find new material uncovered during the essential search of the literature.

When producing material of a specific length, as is invariably the case with coursework, the writer should estimate accurately the number of words per page. This is done by counting the actual number of hand-written words on three pages for example, then dividing by three to find the average page length. Next, the total intended length of the work is divided by the average page length to determine the number of hand-written pages needed to meet the prescribed length. The number of pages for each of the sections should also be estimated.

The coursework, which must be written clearly and attractively, must be 'packaged' and presented well before submission. The first page should be the title page containing various points of information as seen in Example 27.

Example 27 _____

Coursework title page

Smithfield Health College

Year II Diploma in Community Health Care

Student: J.M. Jones

Class: 'Structure of Community Care'

Coursework title: 'Making a clinical assessment is an early part of the treatment process. Discuss'

Lecturer: P.O. Smith

Estimated length: 4500 words

Submission date: 8 December 1993

The second page will be a contents page describing the major parts of the work, as determined in the final structure (see Example 26) along with the initial page number of each part. Example 28 shows how it might look.

Submission

The work should be handed in on or before the submission date using the agreed procedure to guard against loss. Trusting delivery of the work to an unreliable mailing system, or leaving it outside the door of a locked room, is inviting disaster. It is vital to ensure that it is delivered personally and safely, by recorded delivery if mailed, and to retain a photocopy.

The following hints relating to coursework are best read in conjunction with the earlier section relating to examinations and with Chapter 14, 'Dissertations and Theses'.

Example 28 _____

Contents page

Topic	Page number
Introduction	1
Overview of treatment process, position and	
function of clinical assessment	5
...	
...	
...	
Conclusion and general discussion	16
References	19
Bibliography	21

General hints for coursework

- The coursework must be prepared to the prescribed length. Although some examiners accept 10% above or below the requested length, others will deduct marks.
- A formal and recognized reference system must be used *consistently*. If the examiner indicates no preference for a particular system, the writer should follow his or her preference.
- The structure and parts of the coursework answer and the entire piece must be planned as a package. The title and contents page must be planned out carefully.
- All parts of the question must be answered. It is vital that the candidate answer only the question asked. Marks will not be given for material which, however interesting, does not constitute an answer to the question.
- Figures, tables, graphs and other illustrative material should be included if appropriate.
- The candidate should feel free to discuss the proposed answer, in general terms, with the course teacher. This is particularly important if there are any concerns or questions regarding interpretation of the question.
- The course lecturer must be consulted about marking criteria if these have not already been provided. When obtained, they must be studied and the work must comply with the requirements.
- Time should be set aside for undertaking a literature search and review of the subject, and for writing the coursework. It is best to plan to finish the work well ahead of the submission date.
- The work submitted must be clearly written and well presented, typewritten if possible.
- It is vital to ensure that the work is submitted on time, and reaches the appointed person safely. A photocopy must be retained.

Because coursework is prepared without the pressure and constraints of examination-room conditions, examiners expect a high quality of work. This high quality, in terms of content, presentation and structure, is certainly possible if time and energy are invested in preparation. Additionally, coursework preparation is a valuable opportunity for additional learning about the subject and for its revision prior to formal examinations.

If possible, on return of the coursework the allocated marks should be discussed with the teacher, particularly if they are thought to be less than deserved or expected. If the examiner's comments do not make it clear, discussion will establish where the candidate 'went wrong'. In general, coursework well done will attract good marks and give the writer confidence for performing well in formal exams and in clinical, management or teaching roles.

Chapter 10
Books

Although writing a book requires the same range of skills and experience needed to write an article, book authors apply these to a much wider and deeper coverage of the subject matter. All health care professionals should seriously consider using the confidence, knowledge and skill acquired during academic and professional education and subsequent experience to write or edit a textbook.

Whilst all disciplines rely on the use of articles and audio-visual aids for educational and other purposes, the textbook continues to play a key role in the creation and dissemination of professional knowledge. The decision to write or edit a textbook can be arrived at in two distinct ways: the idea can be publisher or writer initiated.

PUBLISHER-INITIATED BOOKS

Publishers and their specialist editors frequently invite health care professionals to identify areas in which textbooks need to be written. For this reason they visit universities, colleges and other places of work to meet staff to discuss and identify gaps in the literature. Gaps in the book literature take a number of forms. A book on the subject might not exist; or existing texts might be out of date. Having established, usually from a number of sources including contacts who provide a form of market research, that a particular book is needed, the publisher will look for someone to write or edit it. Publishers also expect their staff to make and maintain contact with potential book writers and to identify their specialist subject areas.

When a publisher has ascertained, via the firm's specialist/subject editor, that there is a need for a particular book, one or more potential writers may be contacted. If one can be found and the invitation is accepted, the book will probably appear on the bookshelves in two to three years' time. As with writer-initiated books, some of those commissioned by publishers will never be written. In both instances there is a significant failure rate of books which are started but never finished.

WRITER-INITIATED BOOKS

Prospective writers who feel that there is a need for a book on a specific topic are encouraged to contact a publisher and offer to write or edit a book. Such proposals are tentative and do not constitute a firm commitment on either side: much groundwork has to be done before a formal contract stage is reached.

As with writing an article, preparing a book has a number of distinct phases. These are planning, writing and publishing. Example 29 outlines the book publishing process.

PLANNING A BOOK

The major reason for deciding that a new book is required is that it is not but should be available within the existing range of texts. The gap in the literature might be identified by a teacher, a clinician, a manager or a researcher; this underlines the fact that all four groups contribute to producing the professional literature.

Confirming the need

The initial notion that the book is needed but has not yet been written can be confirmed by conducting a thorough literature review to identify existing texts on the subject, and deciding whether or not the subject is adequately covered. The review is then discussed with specialist librarians, with colleagues who work in the subject area, and with the prospective publisher.

Having identified a gap in the literature, it should again be discussed with one or two colleagues, this time with a view to developing and rehearsing arguments which will attract the interest of a potential publisher. Two key issues are of particular interest to the publisher: the need for the book, and the numbers of copies likely to be sold. Book publishing is very costly and is based firmly on commercial considerations.

Having searched the literature and found it to be wanting, and having had the gap in the literature confirmed by colleagues, the next task is to select a publisher.

Selecting a publisher

A look through the bookshelves in a professional library will reveal that a relatively small number of publishers deal with books on health care. The aspiring author should identify three to five publishers who produce good quality texts and publish in their own country. A short letter should be sent to each of the publishers, asking for a copy of the advice and/or guidelines which they have for prospective authors and for a specimen

Example 29 _____

Book publishing process

PLANNING
   Initial idea of need for book
   Confirm need by:
       literature search
       discussing with colleagues
       discussing with teaching staff in the subject area
       discussing with specialist librarian
   Start writing and prepare:
       general description of book (one page)
       general structure of book (chapter list)
       detailed outline of at least first chapter
   Prepare shortlist of possible publishers by:
       examining books in library
       discussing with specialist librarians
       discussing with colleagues
   Contact potential publishers and obtain their:
       guide for authors
       specimen standard contract
   Select a publisher and send:
       covering letter
       material already written
       curriculum vitae
   Receive contract (if publisher wishes to proceed) and:
       clarify unclear points
       ensure equal fairness for author and publisher
       negotiate changes if necessary
       sign contract

WRITING
   Write book by:
       undertaking literature review of subject
       preparing detailed writing timetable
       writing the book (various drafts)
       regularly updating publisher
       submitting the complete manuscript

PUBLISHING
   Receive returned and edited manuscript and:
       agree to or make suggested alterations
       return manuscript to publisher
   Receive proofs and:
       check and recheck the proofs
       clearly indicate corrections
       make minimum amount of changes
       return proofs within agreed timescale
   Receive author's questionnaire and complete and return to publisher
   Receive copies of book and await reviews

copy of their standard contract. At this stage the letter will contain no details of the proposed book. In short, the prospective author is choosing a publisher rather than vice versa.

The replies received may or may not contain additional information that will help in the selection of a publisher. On being contacted in the way described, some publishers may ask for details of the proposed book in order to decide whether or not to accept the proposal, rather than provide the information requested. It is important to persist with the request for publisher's advice and guidelines for authors and a specimen contract. Details of the intended book should not be provided until the publisher has responded, then details of the proposed text should be offered to only one publisher at a time, the one thought best suited to meet the author's needs. In due course a potential publisher is selected and negotiation starts; this usually begins with the publisher asking for more details of the proposal.

Although the type of information requested by publishers will vary, some commonly asked questions are presented to indicate their type and range. The notes following each question have been prepared to illustrate possible replies, and do not form part of the questionnaire sent out by publishers.

QUESTIONNAIRE SENT TO PROSPECTIVE AUTHOR

Q.1   *What is the aim and general purpose of the book?*

Notes   A provisional title and a brief description of the aim of the book must be provided. A draft chapter list, including full chapter titles, will indicate the scope of the book. A few sentences should be included to amplify each chapter title and to provide a one- or two-page outline of the first (introductory) one. The more information a publisher receives about the proposal, the less likely will they be to turn down a good one.

Q.2   *For which readership is the book intended?*

Notes   A clear statement of the intended readership needs to be made. For example, this might be final-year or postgraduate students, or clinicians in a subspecialty. Any other disciplines which might use the book should be mentioned. A small amount of personal market research needs to be undertaken, of clinical and teaching colleagues for example, and should include a sample of comments which are (hopefully) supportive.

Q.3   *Will the book be of particular interest to any undergraduate or postgraduate courses? If so, might it be used as a recommended or reference text?*

Notes   Publishing is a commercial business, and books with a wide potential readership are more attractive to publishers than those with a narrow one. Clearly, a text which may be of use to a small number of highly specialized staff is a less practical proposition for the publisher. Indeed it might be worth considering extending the scope of the book to make it more likely to be used by a wider readership. In order to answer this question well, prospective authors need a good understanding of their discipline generally, not just of their own specialty. If there is any doubt about the range of courses in which the book might be used, this should be discussed with colleagues from other specialties in the discipline and with teaching staff.

Q.4   *What is the anticipated length of the book, and is it likely to include illustrations in the form of photographs, line drawings, tables and figures?*

Notes   Even at this early stage in the development of the book some estimate needs to be made of its possible length. This may be achieved by re-examination of the chapter titles and by roughly estimating the word length of each chapter. Whichever estimate is made, there is room for subsequent revision, but it should be as near as can be achieved (for example to the nearest 10%). A major reason for the publisher needing an answer to this question is a commercial one: the length dictates cost which influences commercial viability. The agreed length will appear in the contract prepared by the publisher.

Q.5   *What is the intended completion date for the manuscript?*

Notes   This depends on the author's personal circumstances, previous experience of writing, and available time. However, in the absence of any better means of making an estimate, two years from the date of signing the contract might be reasonable.

Q.6   *Which other books will compete with the proposed text? If there are competitors, describe why you feel the proposed book to be necessary.*

Notes   Prior to answering this question an actual re-examination of the existing books on the subject is required. Any identified competitors, however weak or strong, must be made known. Publishers realize that a variety of books on a given subject should be available, so acknowledging the existence of competition will not necessarily cause the proposal to be rejected. If any books are identified in response to this question, then details, in the form of a formal reference, photocopy of contents list and price are given to the publisher. Finally, it will be necessary to convince the publisher that, despite the existence of competitors, there is a need for a new book on the subject.

Q.7 *Please give full details of previous professional experience, professional qualifications and all relevant information*

Notes The reply will contain full details of professional experience, qualifications, courses attended, publications, special honours, special interests and membership of any professional committees and societies. This general answer to the question is followed by a more detailed description of those items relating to the subject of the book. For example, if the subject of the book is 'rehabilitation', then all items relating to that area of experience, education and expertise must be discussed in full. An alternative way of answering this question is to refer to an enclosed and suitably adapted curriculum vitae.

Finally the reply to the publisher's questions, the book outline in the form of a chapter list, the curriculum vitae and, preferably, the summary of the introductory chapter, are sent to the selected publisher along with a covering letter.

Publisher's decision

A publisher will weigh up the proposal carefully before deciding whether or not it is a viable one. It will be examined from literary, professional and commercial viewpoints by the publisher's editorial staff, particularly those from the same discipline as the writer of the proposal if the publisher employs such staff. It will also be examined by independent referees to whom the proposal will be sent. The role of the external independent referee in influencing the publisher's decision to accept or reject the proposal is crucial. The types of question the referees will be asked, which are of considerable interest to the prospective author, are discussed fully in Chapter 11.

Publishers tend to encourage modification and improvement generally, and to enable and encourage potential authors to match the proposal to publishing needs rather than reject one prematurely. Proposals are usually only rejected following a long dialogue between the publisher, the writer and external advisors.

If the publisher's reply is negative, reasons for the rejection are usually included. The reply and its implications should be studied carefully prior to considering whether or not another publisher should be contacted. It may be that an otherwise excellent idea is not commercially viable in that the potential readership is too small. The options at this stage are either to offer the proposal to another publisher, to revise it, or to abandon it. The rest of this section will assume that the proposal has been accepted.

THE CONTRACT

The publisher will prepare and send two copies of a standard contract to the author with a request that both be signed and returned for the publisher's signature; one copy is then returned to the author.

The contract constitutes a legal document which is binding on both parties. It must therefore be studied carefully before signing. It is advisable to discuss the contract with someone experienced in the subject, for example another author, or preferably with a literary agent or with the Society of Authors (see Chapter 3).

Contracts vary between publishers, but there are many similarities. Most of the language will be familiar; some will not. In general, contracts are fair and reasonable, but occasionally they contain items which are to the advantage of the publisher at the expense of the author. If thought necessary, the writer should request that changes be made in the contract; it can and should be changed if shown to be unfair, unclear or otherwise inappropriate. If the person negotiating on behalf of the publisher claims that the standard contract cannot be deviated from, this can be challenged if necessary.

A few items that are commonly included in contracts are given below. The list is not, however, exhaustive.

- The *contract title* contains terms such as 'memorandum of agreement' or 'an agreement' followed by the name and address of the author and of the publisher, and the date on which the contract was prepared.
- *Grant of rights* gives the title of the book and indicates that the author grants the publisher exclusive rights to publish and sell the book.
- *Delivery of manuscript* indicates the approximate length of the book, the delivery date for the manuscript, and the number of line drawings, photographs, artwork, etc. If the submission date is not adhered to, or if the manuscript is considered unfit for publication, the publisher reserves the right to rescind the agreement.
- *Additional items* in the form of title page, preface, foreword, contents page, tables, figures and other illustrations, if any, are to be provided by the author.
- The *index* will be prepared by the author, or by a person employed by the author or publisher, and paid by the author.
- *Publication costs* will be met by the publisher.
- *Royalties* are stated in one of several ways, the first being as a percentage of the published price. Thus, if royalties are set at 10% of the published price of £10, the royalty will be £1 per copy sold. The second form of royalty payment is as a percentage of net receipts; that is, a percentage of the price paid to the publisher by the bookseller. Thus, if royalties are set at 10% of net receipts and the publisher receives £6 per book from the bookseller, the royalty per book will be 60p.

  In some instances royalty percentage will increase with the number of copies sold. For example, it might be 10% for the first 3000 copies sold, 12% for the next 3000 copies, and 15%

thereafter; it is reasonable to expect such a sales-related increase.

There may be different royalty rates for overseas sales.

The contract will specify the date on which royalties will be paid, which will be once or twice per year.

- *Free copies* of the book are normally given to the author, six being a typical number.
- *Changes in proofs* are usually allowed and paid for by the publisher to a prescribed maximum. If proof alterations are excessive, costs are usually deducted from royalties. It is essential that proof changes be kept to an *absolute minimum*: making corrections at proof stage is not only very expensive; it may also cause delay and may result in errors being introduced. The author agrees to read, check and correct all proofs, and return them to the publisher within a specified time.
- *Additional editorial work*, if paid for by the publisher, may be deducted from royalties.
- The *author's warranty* includes confirmation by the author that the manuscript is not libellous, defamatory or obscene, and does not infringe existing copyright. Thus, the author takes full legal and personal responsibility for the above aspects of the published text.
- *Advertising* and *production arrangements* are left to the discretion of the publisher: this includes the distribution of free and review copies, and decisions about the form of the binding, jacket and cover of the book. In short, the publisher will take full responsibility for producing and advertising the book and for making it sell.
- *Revisions*, in the form of second and subsequent editions, will be undertaken by the author. In the event of the author's death, or if the author is unwilling or unable to revise, edit and see through the press the second and subsequent editions, the publisher can employ someone to do this, pay them an appropriate fee and deduct that fee from the author's royalties.
- *Keeping the work in print* is the responsibility of the publisher. If a book goes out of print and the publisher decides not to make a reprint or to sign a contract for another edition, it is reasonable for the author and publisher to regard the contract as void and for the author to attempt to have the same or a revised book published elsewhere. Typically, the agreement is ended if the book is out of print and if, within nine months after notice in writing from the author, the publisher has not reprinted further copies and placed them on the market.
- *Competing publications*, that is those that affect prejudicially the sale of the work, should not be published by the publisher during the term of the contract. Equally, the author agrees not to publish or to furnish to any other publisher any work of a nature which is likely to affect prejudicially the sale of the work.
- *Copyright infringement*. The publisher will take action in the

author's name against such infringement. The net proceeds of such a claim will be divided equally between the author and the publisher.

WRITING THE BOOK

The time taken to write a book varies considerably depending on the amount of previous preparation, the author's writing skills and the extent to which the ideas for the book have developed. Typically, the manuscript submission date will be two years from the signing of the contract, but publishers allow some flexibility.

At this stage it is necessary to begin to prepare a firm timetable of events for writing the book. For example, if there are 12 major sections or chapters, the time allocation might be as follows: three months for further planning of the work, for research and making detailed notes about each part; 18 months for writing the 12 chapters, and three months for putting the book together and thoroughly checking every item in it.

PUBLISHER'S GUIDE FOR AUTHORS

Most publishers prepare a guide for their authors. If this has not already been obtained it should be requested. Understandably, the guide is fairly general and relates to structure, presentation and some aspects of style rather than to content. The following items are typical of those provided by a publishing house in its author's guide.

- *Presentation of manuscript*. The final copy must be typed on one side of A4 paper, using double spacing and leaving a 3.8 cm (1½ in) margin on all sides. Three copies should be prepared, the top and second copy being sent to the publisher and the third retained. The pages in the manuscript must be numbered in sequence throughout, including appendices and reference list. All tables and figures must be referred to in the text at a point very close to where they are to be presented. The agreed chapter and manuscript length must be adhered to. All minor corrections must be legible and clearly made in the text or indicated in the margin. Lengthy corrections must be typed on a separate A4 sheet and their place and page number indicated.
- *Style*. Advice on the use of abbreviations, symbols, numbers and means of referring to figures and tables may be given in the guide. For example, it might be to use 'per cent' in the text but the symbol '%' in the tables. Advice may also be given on the use of drug names, the approved name being most commonly required. Points of style not referred to in this section, but which need to be discussed, must be raised with the publisher.

- *Use of italics.* The use of italics, or of underlining if the typewriter does not have an italic facility, should be explained in the guide. For example, it may state that foreign words, titles of books in journals and quotations should be italicized.
- *Specimen presentation.* A short example of how material should be presented may be included. This will probably be used to highlight important points and problem areas.
- *Illustrations.* Clear instructions as to the use and location of illustrations including photographs, line drawings or other types of illustration must be obtained. For example, it is usual for each illustration to be produced on a separate page at the end of the manuscript rather than incorporated into the manuscript text. Most publishers have specific requirements and are unable to use material which does not meet them.
- *Headings.* These are used to make the text more readable and visually attractive. In addition to the chapter heading, three or four subsidiary headings may be used. Whether or not the typewriter has the facility to print headings of different sizes, it is normal practice to indicate the grade or weight of the heading in the left margin. For example, if the heading is the major or primary heading, then the encircled number 1 or letter A is placed in the margin to the left of that heading. Similarly, if the heading is the lowest rank or grade of four, then an encircled number 4 or letter D will be placed in the margin to the left.
- *References.* Authors will be given a clear indication of the reference style to be used in the manuscript. The guide will also contain some examples of how the references should be cited in the text and presented in the reference list.
- *Footnotes.* Footnotes are generally discouraged. If they are essential, they should be placed on a separate sheet at the end of the manuscript with an indication of the page number on which they should be inserted.
- *Proofs.* A brief indication of the arrangement for proofreading the manuscript may be included. Alternatively, detailed instructions regarding the proofreading process may be provided along with the proofs.
- *Index.* Although the need for constructing an index may be mentioned at this stage, serious work on it cannot begin until after the completion of the manuscript. It is usual for full instructions regarding the compilation of an index to be sent at a later stage. (See also Chapter 12.)

WRITING

The principles discussed elsewhere in this book, for example in relation to an article or research report, also apply to writing a book. The content and structure of individual chapters require attention as does the relationship of one chapter to all the others. The individual chapters together constitute the general structure of the book and so must be placed in the best possible sequence.

There are features of a book's structure which are unique to it and which are rarely found in other areas of writing. Although these additional items need not be written until work has ended on all chapters, they may be referred to in the text.

Foreword

Many books contain a foreword. This is a short introductory section at the front of the book and is written by an authority on the subject who has been invited to do so. The foreword is traditionally written in such a way as to draw the reader's attention to the book's strengths.

Preface or prologue

The preface or prologue is a short introductory section written by the author. Although its major function is to present the aim and intent of the text in a general manner, it also frequently incorporates the acknowledgement of assistance from those whose help made the book possible. Otherwise, the acknowledgements occupy their own section.

Dedication

On occasion the author will dedicate the book to a person, institution or belief. The style of the dedication will vary considerably but might take one of the following forms:

'This book is dedicated to my husband and family'
   or
'This book is dedicated to my teachers'
   or
'This book is dedicated to the future development of my profession'.

Other elements of the structure which are considered to be 'optional' and about which decisions about inclusion need to be made include: a bibliography, a glossary, reading lists and practical exercises.

PUBLISHING

When the manuscript has been submitted to the publisher, it will be sent to one or more reviewers. It is then edited and any queries that arise are discussed with the author. Unless there are exceptional circumstances, the manuscript is not returned to the author at this stage. More commonly it is returned in the form of galley or page proofs. In any event the book will be returned to the author at some stage for detailed checking. This tedious task of manuscript proofreading requires considerable time, effort and accuracy. The job of the author is to check and recheck every word, sentence and heading of the work to make absolutely sure that everything is correct in meaning, style and presentation. When this is complete, the manuscript or proof is returned to the publisher with the relevant corrections clearly marked. This subject is discussed more fully in Chapter 12. One point, however, that should be borne in mind at all stages is the need to keep the publisher informed in advance of any change of address (personal and professional) and of any extended absences from these addresses. It serves no purpose to have manuscripts or proofs – or, worse, a royalty cheque – sitting on an empty desk or stuck at the post office in search of the addressee.

Although publishers have the sole responsibility for publishing the text and for maximizing its commercial success, they will look to the author for assistance in relation to the latter function. Because authors are particularly knowledgeable about the subject of the text, they may be asked for information that will help in promotion. This might, for example, include suggestions as to the journals to which review copies of the book should be sent. Authors can also help by providing the names of professional groups, conferences or societies who should be informed about the work. They should be prepared to participate in the production of publicity for the book by providing information about personal experience, background and interest in its subject.

EDITING A BOOK

An increasing number of books are edited rather than written by one or two authors. The advantages of being an editor rather than an author are that the work is shared with other contributors, and that a much wider range of expertise is included in the authorship of the book. In this context the function of the editor is to contact a number of writers, each of whom will write one or more chapters of the book. The editor, who will also contribute to the book, plays a major part in coordinating the efforts of all the authors, ensuring the overall quality and continuity of the work and making decisions about the sequence of chapters. An editor will also examine and, if necessary, edit all contributions to ensure that they are consistent in quality, style and level of presentation. Occasionally an editor will have to find a replacement for a writer who finds, sometimes very close to the submission date, that a writing commitment cannot be met.

As with multiauthor books, ones with more than one editor will have an editor who is regarded as being the senior (first named) one. The decision as to who will be the senior editor *must* be taken very early on in the project. The senior editor is the person who generates the idea for the book, contacts additional co-editors, communicates with the publisher, and generally has the major responsibility for coordinating the work of others and for ensuring delivery of the manuscript on time.

Contract

Each contributor requires a brief contract, usually in the form of a letter from the publisher, with details such as chapter title(s), length, submission date and royalty payment. It is usual for the editor to decide on the level of royalty offered to them, and for that to be a pro-rata share of royalties after the deduction of, for example, 30% payable to the editor. Thus, if the royalty is 10% of the published price of a book selling for £10 per copy and there are ten chapters, royalty distribution will be: editor, 30 pence per copy sold; contributors of each chapter, 7 pence per copy sold.

When producing a book as an author or editor, a good working relationship should be formed and maintained with the appropriate member of the publisher's staff. Invariably the publishing company will assign one of its staff to work with the author or editor, this relationship continuing from start to finish. The author or editor should feel free to get in touch with the publisher or assigned member of staff if there are any questions regarding the production of the book.

Any difficulties must be reported immediately to the publisher. For example, if agreed deadlines cannot be met because of illness or other similar reasons, it is vital that the publisher be contacted immediately.

Whether as editor or author, having a book published is a formidable task which, in addition to contributing to the professional literature, gives a considerable amount of personal satisfaction. It is important to enjoy the complimentary reviews, and to learn from constructive criticism so that the next edition can be improved.

Chapter 11
Publishing Consultancies

Among other publishing-related opportunities available to writers is consultancy work. Although poorly paid or indeed sometimes unpaid, the personal rewards for this type of work are considerable. The need for health care professionals to be recruited to this advisory role results from the need of some publishing companies to employ specialists, on either a part-time or ad hoc basis. Such an arrangement also helps publishers keep abreast of developments and changes within the professions which they serve.

Traditionally, consultancy work has resulted from individuals being contacted by publishers. Now, however, new and established publishers of books and journals encourage members of all professions to get in touch and discuss possible contributions.

A number of qualities are required by those who are involved in consultancy work. A thorough knowledge of the subject matter of the work is certainly necessary. Honesty and integrity are of considerable importance, bearing in mind that the material received at a pre-publication stage is highly confidential. Similarly, the consultant may have to give a full and frank, positive or negative opinion of the quality of work of others. The consultant is frequently asked to stick to a fixed deadline, and should only accept work which can be completed in the agreed time. The ability to review objectively the quality of a given piece is essential and requires thorough familiarity with the subject in order that criticism can be constructive. A clear and succinct writing style is also required.

A selection of the more commonly used consultancies are presented along with notes on what might be expected by a publisher. The reader should bear in mind that there is considerable variation in the requirements of different publishers.

BOOKS

Book publishers are the main consumers of consultancy services involving book proposals, submitted manuscripts and sometimes published books.

Book proposals

Having received details of a proposed book from a prospective author, the publisher will first do market research and, when this is positive and indicates a need for the book, will then undertake a detailed discussion with a consultant who will act as a 'referee'.

The following questions are typical of those that may be sent to a referee along with details of the proposal. The notes following each question have been included for readers of this text, and would not form part of the questionnaire sent out by the publisher.

Questionnaire sent to book proposal referee

Q.1 *Is there a need for this type of book?*

Notes   Publishers are aware of the universal scope of health care and of the need for their books to have an international appeal. Some attempt should be made to answer this question in relation to an international readership.

If books on the subject already exist, including those published overseas, the value of an additional one on the subject is commented on. If existing books have deficiencies which the proposed one does not have, then this is made known to the publisher.

As with all other questions, this one will already have been answered by the potential author who proposed the book. However, the publisher is interested in obtaining a second, and perhaps a third and fourth, assessment of the worth of the proposal, that is independent. Such is the high financial cost of commercial failure that publishers do much to ensure, as far as possible, that only commercially viable proposals reach book stage.

Q.2 *What are the major competitors to this book?*

Notes   Publishers look to the referee to use knowledge of the literature on the subject and to inform them of existing books on the subject or of books that are known to be in preparation. If known, full reference to those works should be given together with general details of their contents, and a comparison must be made between the existing books and the one being proposed.

Q.3 *Would you recommend publication of this book?*

Notes   The publisher is looking for more than a 'Yes' or 'No' answer to this; whichever answer is given is argued and justified. Many referees find answering this question difficult, particularly since the answer will have considerable impact on the career and literary aspirations of a fellow professional. However, it is important to bear in mind that a final decision is taken by the publisher following consultation with a number of independent referees. In short, any decision to accept or reject a proposal is a collective one.

Q.4 *Who might buy this book?*

Notes The groups, obvious and less obvious, who might find the book of use must be indicated. The potential primary readers (those for whom the book was obviously intended) must be identified as should any secondary reader groups (those who will have some interest in it).

The specific courses for which the book might be used as either a major text or as supplementary reading should be stated if possible.

Q.5 *What is the size of the potential readership?*

Notes Some estimate can be made of the total number of readers on the following basis. If the book is potentially suitable for use as a major text for postregistration students attending courses relating to the care of the elderly, for example, all schools offering the course might be asked, by the referee or the publisher, for their annual student intake. Similarly, if the book is directed at a particular staff grade, it may be possible to establish the size of that group from existing statistical material such as that published by government departments. However, rather than specify the potential number of readers, it is usually more appropriate and possible to describe the group and leave the publisher to establish or estimate its size. Such a description might be: 'All undergraduate students in the discipline to which the proposal relates.'

When it is impossible to obtain figures for an estimate of the potential readership, the publisher should be told. If an estimate is made, reasons for arriving at that particular figure should be given.

Q.6 *Do you have any suggestions for improving this proposal?*

Notes Any obvious omissions from the proposal are commented on, as are any unnecessary inclusions. Publishers are *very* keen to receive well argued, independent and constructive professional criticism. If a sample chapter is included, then comments can be made on writing style, use of references, readability, presentation and scholarship. Although these aspects will be obvious to an established publisher, a second opinion is always valued.

Q.7 *Can you name other experts in this subject area?*

Notes The publisher may wish to use the services of additional referees but may need help in finding suitable people. Where possible the referee should suggest the names of others who can then be approached by the publisher.

Q.8   *Are the professional experience, qualifications and background of the proposal writer appropriate to the book?*

Notes   It is important that a full curriculum vitae accompany the proposal in order that an opinion can be expressed regarding the professional, academic and experiential suitability of the proposed author. If the proposal has been written by an acknowledged expert in the field, their suitability should be less difficult to gauge than if the writer is relatively unknown.

Q.9   *Are there any other points you wish to make?*

Notes   Here any additional relevant comments which have not been covered in the questionnaire should be included.

Q.10   *May we disclose your identity?*

Notes   Some publishers may wish to disclose the identity of referees; most prefer to preserve anonymity. However, should they wish to disclose the name of the referee to the proposal writer, it is necessary to obtain the referee's permission to do so.

The preceding sample questionnaire which publishers send to referees may also be of value to those preparing a proposal for submission to a publisher. Having established, on the basis of a proposal and perhaps a sample chapter, that a book is required, is likely to be of a high enough standard and appears to be commercially viable, the publisher will then prepare a contract inviting the prospective author to work on a complete manuscript. When the manuscript is eventually submitted, the publisher will, in addition to having it examined by 'in house' staff, send it to one or more referees. The purpose of this second refereeing process is to establish that the content, level and quality of the text are as promised in the proposal. Entering into a contract with a publisher does not guarantee that the manuscript will be published.

Submitted manuscripts

Although the guidelines sent to those refereeing submitted manuscripts vary from publisher to publisher, the basic questions are similar.

Publishers do not usually ask referees to examine grammar or typographical quality of the manuscript as these are publishing criteria and are taken care of during the publishing process. It is helpful, however, to bring misspelling of scientific terms to their attention. The referee is normally asked for a professional assessment of the content of the work and of its general readability, and whether or not the presentation is of an acceptable professional level.

As publishers should not make known the name of the referee

without prior permission, so they should not use the favourable comments of the referee for promotional or advertising purposes without prior consent.

Questionnaire sent to manuscript referee

Q.1   *Is the work readable and interesting?*

Notes   Here, the publisher is asking for the opinion of the referee in the role of an informed reader and consumer of professional literature.

Q.2   *Is the material accurate and well organized?*

Notes   Professional skills and knowledge are required to answer this question. Experience of using similar texts will help the reviewer to comment on whether its organization is logical for its intended purpose. The general layout of the material in the manuscript may also be commented on although this is an area in which the publisher's editorial staff have special expertise.

Q.3   *Is the level of the material right?*

Notes   Books are usually aimed at a particular readership, students or trained staff for example, or are meant for a general rather than a specialist readership. The level at which the material is presented must coincide with its prospective readership.

Q.4   *Is the author well informed?*

Notes   The referee is being asked to make a professional judgement about whether the author is well informed in relation to the subject of the book. Obviously, expertise in the subject area is the prime reason for being invited to referee the manuscript.

Q.5   *Who might use the book?*

Notes   The relevance of the book to professional training and continuing education, whether the referee would recommend it, and the course, groups and specialties for which the book would be most suitable constitute the answer to this question.

Q.6   *Is the subject fully covered?*

Notes   The extent to which the subject matter of the book is fully or inadequately dealt with is stated here. If a shift of emphasis within all or part of the book is needed, this is brought to the attention of the publisher.

Published books

Publishers will occasionally consult referees about books that have already been published. For example, if an existing one is going into a further edition, the publisher may ask one or more experts in the subject area to comment on aspects of it. Depending on referees' responses, the publisher may or may not suggest that the author make changes. Another example of this type of consultancy is when a book is to be released in a country other than the one in which it was originally published. In this instance the referee will make a detailed examination of the content, presentation and language of the book to determine whether changes are required prior to its release in the 'new' country. An example of this type of work is when a book published in and for the United States of America requires to be anglicized prior to its release in the British market.

GENERAL CONSULTANCY

A few publishers may pay one or more consultants an annual retention fee for general advice. They meet the consultant three or four times a year to discuss new projects and subjects requiring book coverage and to report on changes in methods and approach. Such consultants are also expected to provide names and to verify the abilities of potential authors and referees.

If the volume of work given to the consultant exceeds the level of annual payment made by the publisher, then additional payments may be made on an ad hoc basis.

JOURNAL REFEREEING

A number of journals have a panel of referees to whom they send submitted article manuscripts prior to accepting them for publication. Although the specific remit of this type of referee may vary slightly from journal to journal, the same types of question are usually asked.

Questionnaire sent to article referee

Q.1   *Does the manuscript comply with the journal's guide to contributors?*

Notes   The referee examines such aspects as length, use of references and general content, and ensures that the manuscript complies with the requirements of the journal.

Q.2 *Is the factual material in the manuscript accurate?*

Notes Facts such as drug doses, physiological values, laws and statistical material are checked for accuracy.

Q.3 *Does the quality and general standard of the manuscript meet the requirements of the journal?*

Notes The experience of the referee, combined with a knowledge of the journal's standards, will enable a judgement to be made as to the quality of the manuscript.

Q.4 *Is the material topical, original and up to date?*

Notes Here the referee relies largely on personal experience and knowledge of professional literature relating to the subject of the manuscript.

As with books, the identity of referees is confidential and revealed only with the explicit permission of the referee. In some instances there may be a distinct advantage in asking the manuscript author to contact the referee to discuss how the material might be adjusted to meet the requirements of the journal. However, dialogue usually takes place between the journal editor and the author.

Authors of submitted manuscripts appreciate that the job of the referee is to submit an honest and objective appraisal of the work. On receiving a referee's negative comments it would be inappropriate for the author to try to establish, or still worse guess, the identity of the referee. A guess is liable to be wrong and can seriously damage professional relationships.

EDITORIAL PANEL MEMBER

A number of journals, often headed by a member of the profession which the journal serves, use the services of consultants who constitute the editorial panel. These consultants, who may be paid or unpaid, are used for purposes which vary from journal to journal. They may act as book reviewers or article referees or may be asked to meet the editor periodically to discuss the editorial policies of the journal. This arrangement ensures that a strong relationship exists between the publisher and the profession for which it publishes.

Although those journals with a large editorial staff have less need for this type of arrangement, more specialized journals with a smaller circulation depend heavily on the contribution and input of its editorial panel.

BECOMING A PUBLISHING CONSULTANT

While the types of consultant previously discussed are often recruited by publishers, there is no reason why individuals interested in taking on such a role should not get in touch with a publisher and offer to make their services available. Clearly, the terms of such an arrangement would need to be fully discussed before either party makes a final commitment.

Information should be provided to the publisher by anyone who wishes to get involved in consultancy work. This should include a full and detailed curriculum vitae and a clear statement of the type of consultancy work being sought. For example, if writing to a journal and requesting consideration for appointment to its panel of book reviewers, details of particular specialist areas in which review work is sought should be given.

Chapter 12
Manuscript Checking, Proofreading and Indexing

Having prepared the final draft of the manuscript, whether this be for an article, a chapter or a book, it must now be thoroughly checked before submission to the publisher. At this stage the content, presentation, layout and accuracy are given a final inspection. Although radical changes are unlikely at this stage, a number of minor alterations may be necessary. If the corrections are minor, as is usually the case, they can be corrected without retyping. If major, the manuscript must be retyped, then checked again. All corrections and alterations must be incorporated clearly into the typescript. It might be prudent to try out the alterations and corrections in pencil in the available space before using ink.

CHECKING

Pagination changes

Until the manuscript is about to be sent to the publisher, all page numbers should be in pencil. The advantage of this is that the numbers can be changed if pages (or folios as the publisher will prefer to call them to distinguish them from the printed pages) are added to or removed from the total length of the work.

If the folio numbers have already been typed on to the manuscript and changes have to be made, the following method can be used. If folios are added, their numbers become continuous with the existing one that precedes the additional ones. For example, if two new folios are to be inserted immediately after folio 9, those added are numbered 9a and 9b. In the bottom margin of folio 9, an encircled note stating 'Followed by folios 9a and 9b' will draw attention to the additions. If folios have to be removed from the manuscript, the numbers on the original folios are left unchanged but a note is added on the preceding page. For example, if folios 11 and 12 are removed, then an encircled note in the bottom margin of folio 10 stating 'Folios 11 and 12 have been removed' (or 'Folio 13 follows') will draw attention to the omissions. Finally, in the covering letter to the publisher that accompanies the manuscript, attention should be drawn to additional or omitted pages.

References

A common error in works containing references to previously published works is the failure of the references in the text to match *exactly* those in the reference list at the end. When checking the manuscript, each reference must be cross-matched with its entry in the reference list. Thus, if Pink (1993) is found in the text, its presence must be checked in the reference list. As each reference in the text is located in the reference list, a temporary mark should be made in pencil against the item in the list. When the manuscript has been read in full, all items in the reference list should have a pencil mark against them, confirming that all in the list have actually been cited in the text. Finally, the opportunity must be taken to make a final check on all aspects of the bibliographical detail of the references in the reference list.

Corrections

Example 30 shows how part of a manuscript requiring corrections might appear. It is followed by the same material (Example 31) which has been set in type to demonstrate how the corrections have been incorporated by the typesetter.

Example 30

Manuscript requiring corrections

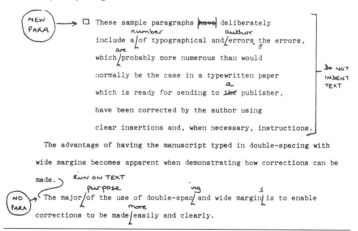

When checking the manuscript, it is easy, bearing in mind that it will have been read many times before, to overlook obvious errors. When making the final check, it is useful to read the work aloud to detect errors in meaning as well as typographical errors. Ideally, a colleague should listen to the reading.

No matter how well the manuscript has been checked, errors of style, content and presentation will be picked up by the publisher's copy editor. However, the publisher's printer may introduce errors when transcribing the manuscript into print, that is, when typesetting. For this reason, the publisher submits proofs to the author for proofreading and correcting.

Example 31 _____

Corrected manuscript

These sample paragraphs deliberately include a number of typographical and author errors. The errors, which are probably more numerous than would normally be the case in a typewritten paper which is ready for sending to a publisher, have been corrected by the author using clear insertions and, when necessary, instructions.

The advantage of having the manuscript typed in double-spacing with wide margins becomes apparent when demonstrating how corrections can be made. The major purpose of the use of double-spacing and wide margins is to enable corrections to be made more easily and clearly.

_____

PROOFREADING

The publisher sends proof copies of the manuscript to the writer for proofreading, that is, checking for typographical or factual errors. Although a minimal amount of other alterations to the work may be permitted at this stage, these can be costly to the publisher who may hold the writer financially responsible if such alterations exceed a predetermined percentage of the total cost of typesetting the manuscript.

On receipt of the proof copy it is compared with the original type-script, a copy of which will have been retained by the author. It should be noted that the author will not usually have details of the marks made by the copy editor. It is difficult to overemphasize the need for concentration, accuracy and care when reading proofs. Ideally, the proofs should be read aloud to a colleague who can compare the material with the original manuscript. When checking this way, it is necessary that everything be read and compared: every full stop, comma, capital letter, spelling of person and place names, every dash, and so on. In short, *everything* that appears on the proof page must be checked in fine detail.

The corrections made on the proofs by the author may take one of two forms, depending on instructions received from the publisher. Occasionally, the publisher will simply request that clear and legible corrections be made in the margin. Alternatively, and more usually, the publisher will provide a list of recognized proof correction marks (see Example 32) which are used in the margin and text to indicate items for correction. Although the proof correction marks used by different publishers may vary slightly, those shown in Example 32 (used by the

Example 32

Proof correction marks

Any errors in this proof which have been noticed by the printer's reader have been marked in green. If you see any more printer's errors, please mark them in red; there is no charge for correcting these mistakes. For your own alterations, please use black or blue or any colour other than green or red. Please use the proof correction marks shown below for all alterations and corrections.

Instruction to printer	Textual mark	Marginal mark
Leave unchanged	. . . under matter to remain	⊘
Insert in text the matter indicated in the margin	⅄	New matter followed by ⅄
Delete	⊢⊣ through matter to be deleted	ℰ
Delete and close up	⟨⊃ through matter to be deleted	ℰ
Substitute character or substitute part of one or more word(s)	/ through letter or ⊢⊣ through word	New letter or new word
Change to italics	___ under matter to be changed	⌴⌴⌴
Change to capitals	≡ under matter to be changed	≡
Change to small capitals	= under matter to be changed	=
Change to bold type	∿∧ under matter to be changed	∿∿∿
Change to bold italic	≈ under matter to be changed	⌴⌴⌴
Change to lower case	Encircle matter to be changed	≢
Change italic to upright type	[As above]	⌴⌴
Insert 'superior' character	/ through character or ⅄ where required	⅄ under character, e.g. ⅄
Insert 'inferior' character	[As above]	⅃ over character, e.g. ⅃
Insert full stop	[As above]	⊙
Insert comma	[As above]	?
Insert single quotation marks	[As above]	⅄ and/or ⅄
Insert double quotation marks	[As above]	⅄ and/or ⅄
Insert hyphen	[As above]	⊢⊣
Start new paragraph	⌐	⌐
No new paragraph	⊃	⊃
Transpose	⌐⌐	⌐⌐
Close up	linking ⊃ letters	◌
Insert space between letters	⌶ between letters affected	⅄
Insert space between words	⅄ between words affected	⅄
Reduce space between letters	⌶ between letters affected	⌃
Reduce space between words	⌃ between words affected	⌃

BLACKWELL SCIENTIFIC PUBLICATIONS

publisher of this book) are typical of many. In this example the publisher has requested that the author use different colours of ink to indicate printer's errors and personal alterations. This distinction is made to enable the publisher to avoid having to pay for the correction of printer's errors.

The material in the left-hand column of Example 32 ('Instruction to printer') is *not* entered on the proof. Only the symbols in the middle and right-hand columns are used. Whether or not proof marks are to be used, the important point is that the author and the publisher have the same understanding of the symbols used.

Having sent proofs to the author for checking, the publisher will wish to have them returned as quickly as possible, within two weeks for example. Because of the time scale within which the publisher is now working it is essential that *every* effort be made to comply with such a request. If there is any anticipated delay, due to planned holidays for example, then this must be made known to the publisher well in advance and alternative arrangements must be made.

INDEXING

An index is an alphabetical list of names or subjects, together with the page number on which they appear in the text. Although the index can be prepared by a professional indexer and paid for by the author, some writers prefer to produce their own. If it is prepared by a professional indexer, whether hired by the author or by the publisher, it is essential that the author read and check the index manuscript. The author will wish to correct any errors in the index and add to its general quality by virtue of personal knowledge of the subject matter. Professional indexers' fees can be expensive and the author's knowledge of the text is a considerable advantage in personally preparing the index. Many writers therefore undertake this task themselves and do so successfully. In such cases it is important to seek the publisher's advice, and request any publishing guides to, or list of, literature on index preparation.

The index, which is normally only necessary in books, is placed at the end of the publication. There are two commonly used types of index: an author index (which is not always necessary) and a subject index. These two types may be combined to form an author and subject index. However, for the sake of illustration they will be discussed separately here.

Author index

An author index may be necessary if the book contains a large number of references to other people's published works, and if it is thought that readers are likely to want to locate references to the work of a specific writer. A reader of the book may wish to establish on which page or pages citations of the work(s) of a particular author appear. The numbers of those pages will be set against the name of the author in the index where they are alphabetically listed. Many texts combine their author and subject index; others make no index reference to authors cited in the book but rely on the reference list for such information retrieval. Example 33 shows how an author index might look.

Example 33

Sample author index

Ambrose, P.	34, 45
Clark, D.	99
Krankler, J.	2, 89
Poult, L.	17
Serf, G.	5, 34, 66
West, H.	45
Yalter, E.	98, 104

Subject index

The subject index is an alphabetical list using entries, subentries and subsubentries to identify the contents of a book and to direct the reader to the relevant pages. It is clearly much more specific and detailed than the list of contents placed at the front of the book, and will include items of relevance which are mentioned either briefly or extensively in the text.

Because writing the index cannot be completed until after page proofs have been received from the publisher, the task is often left until the last minute. To avoid a late rush, work on the index should be started as early as possible. For example, the retained copy of the manuscript sent to the publisher can be used to highlight those items likely to be included in the index. These can then be transferred to alphabetically lettered index cards or, better still, can be typed into a word processor in alphabetical sequence. If the card system is used, the cards are subsequently sorted into alphabetical sequence, arranged into entries, subentries and sub-subentries, then typed up. In fact the index can be prepared in this way before receipt of proofs from the publisher, although the page numbers on which items appear can only be added when the page proofs are received.

Index entries must include, and preferably begin with, a noun and must be followed by the page number(s) on which the entries appear. The use of capital letters in an index will vary from publisher to publisher. Some may prefer to use lower case for all entries that do not have capitals in the text while others will accept each main entry beginning with a capital letter (the style used in this book). Entries may be further divided into subentries, and possibly sub-subentries. For example the entry 'Community care' might have the subentry 'location of' which in turn has the subentries (known as sub-subentries) 'home', 'nursing home' and 'residential home'. In all cases any subentries should always be lower case unless capitalized in the text, for example 'Department of Health'. Example 34 shows how such an index might look.

Example 34 _____

Sample subject index

Activities of daily living	89, 107
Association of Community Care Clinicians	34, 56, 89
Community care	45–7, 68, 99
Department of Health	75
location of	69–78
home	70
nursing home	73–4
residential home	77
Rehabilitation	4, 45–6, 174

The question of indexing must be discussed with the publisher early and decisions must be made as to whether it will be a subject index only, separate subject and author indexes, or a combined subject and author index. It is necessary at this stage to decide who will prepare the index, the author or a professional indexer, and if the latter how they will be recruited and paid.

Chapter 13
Research Reports

A major feature of all pieces of research is the written report. This requirement exists whether or not the report is to be published. Although writing a report is only one part of the research process, it is a particularly important and challenging one. The purpose of this chapter is not to discuss the research process, only that part of it relating to writing up the report.

The preparation of a report will be necessary irrespective of the purpose for which the research was undertaken. The same principles apply to an informal small-scale study, to a Doctor of Philosophy thesis, and to a large-scale project undertaken by a team of researchers.

It is often said that health care research is rarely read and less frequently implemented. This criticism may, in part, result from the fact that many research reports are badly written. Unless reports are written in a readable and meaningful form, their potential effectiveness is much reduced.

Many researchers experience difficulty in preparing a written description of their work. This discussion is intended to minimize these difficulties and should be used *in addition* to any instructions offered by the institution which has commissioned the research, or to the requirements of the institution awarding the research degree. If the report is to be published, it must be written in compliance with the requirements of the publisher.

STRUCTURE

The writing-up phase of the research process can run parallel with all other phases of the process, or may occur at the end. In either case it is widely accepted that a specific part of the 'time budget' should be set aside for this purpose. A useful starting point is to consider the structure of the research process which in turn constitutes the structure of the report. Although there is no blueprint for the structure of the former, that being influenced by the research design used by the researcher, the report will reflect whichever structure and design are used. The remainder of this chapter is based on one type of research process structure and design, whilst acknowledging that there are others.

Introduction

A general introduction to the subject of the report should include a discussion of its importance and of the need for it to be researched. The research problem must be clearly identified, as must be the thinking process that initiated the research.

The relationship of the work to past, current and future projects must be made clear. The background and experience of the researcher are often included here to place the work in a personal context. After reading the introduction the reader should be quite clear about the nature and purpose of the research.

Aims of the research

A detailed discussion of the aims of the research, including operational definitions of the main terms in the title, should then follow. The research question(s) which the study intends to answer must be presented. Some but by no means all researchers state and then test research hypotheses. The aims of the research are then listed in a concise form at the end of their more general discussion.

Literature review

A detailed presentation, review and analysis of previously published relevant literature should then be given. This should demonstrate how the current research was influenced by, and will develop from, published literature, some of which will be research based and some not. The purpose of the review is to inform the reader of relevant literature and to state how it relates to the present study. Literature that is supportive to *and* that which disagrees with the research being reported is included.

This part of the report will be much more easily prepared if all references previously collected are recorded on alphabetically filed index cards or on a computing system. It is *absolutely essential* that a well organized record be kept of all references. See Chapter 5 for a discussion of how to incorporate references into written work, and Chapters 6 and 7 for a discussion of how to search and review the literature.

Research design

The term 'research design' is used to describe the overall research approach to be used. A variety of designs can be used, either singly or in some instances in combination; examples include qualitative and quantitative designs, and grounded theory, experimental, action, historical and evaluation research designs. The design of a study, which is not to be confused with the data collection method which is part of the design, must be described in detail. The report should include a clear justification for the choice of design(s).

This section must also include a detailed description of, and justification for, the data collection method(s) to be used; examples include interview, observation and questionnaire. It should also describe, in detail, *every* step of the means by which data are collected. This description will enable readers to understand the data collection methods, judge their suitability, and be able to repeat (replicate) them if necessary. The validity and reliability of all data collection instruments must be discussed, as must anticipated problems.

The population and method of sample selection and any sampling techniques used must be described. If experimental methods feature in the research, they should be reported in detail.

Ethical considerations

The length of this section will depend on whether or not the research is likely to raise any ethical issues. If no such issues were anticipated, and none has emerged during the research, this part of the report can be short; otherwise they must be discussed fully as must the steps taken to deal with them.

Assurances regarding confidentiality and anonymity are a common feature of many research projects. The means by which these are made to actual or potential respondents should be described, as should the methods employed to ensure that the assurances are adhered to.

Entry to the research site

Most research studies are dependent on obtaining permission from individuals, committees or managers to enter a site for the purpose of collecting research data. Details of how this has been achieved, including correspondence with research and ethics committees, should be covered.

Data collection

This section describes how research data were actually obtained. Any difficulties experienced during this phase, particularly if they affected the study, are acknowledged and discussed.

If this phase constitutes or includes a pilot study, its outcome in terms of adequacy or otherwise must be included as must details of any resultant changes in the research method.

Data analysis

Collected data must be described, analysed and presented in a clear and unambiguous form. If data are subjected to statistical analysis, the statistical test chosen must be described.

Conclusions and discussion

The major aim of the closing section of a research report is to draw conclusions from the study while bearing in mind any limitations. The inclusion of informed opinion is not merely permissible; it is essential provided that the reader can distinguish it from research-based fact.

The discussion must enable speculation about the meaning of the findings, recognition of the limitations of the study and suggestions for future research in the subject area. No new material in the form of research data should be introduced in this section.

Finally, a brief summary of the major findings of the study must be presented.

In addition to the structure, other aspects of the report should be considered before and during the actual research and whilst the report is being written. The report must not be developed haphazardly. During its construction the following two points must be borne in mind:

Reason (Why is the report being written?)
  and
Readership and language (Who will be reading the report, and what form of language will be best understood?)

REASONS FOR PRODUCING A RESEARCH REPORT

Irrespective of how many or how few people have an interest in the findings of a piece of research, it is necessary to prepare a written report of it. Apart from providing a permanent record of the work, the actual task of writing up adds much to the researcher's understanding of it and helps avoid the use of generalities which are often a feature of verbal description. Many reports are written to comply with a condition of the commissioning institution or of a grant-awarding body, for example. If the research is undertaken in order to obtain a higher degree, producing a report in the form of a thesis will be necessary.

In terms of a more general readership, the report has two major purposes: to make the findings available, and to give details of the research design used, including the data collection methods.

The full details of the findings of a research report should include those that supported any hypotheses or expectations, those that contradicted them, and those that were inconclusive. When possible, raw data, or liberal samples of them, should be included in addition to the more frequently used summaries of data.

Following the presentation of data (fact) there should be a full discussion of the meaning and implications of the research findings. This should include input which draws on personal experience and knowledge of the subject (opinion). In this concluding section the data should be interpreted and used to increase knowledge of the subject, and should give direction to further related research.

In some instances only part of a report may be published. For example, an article might contain a summary of the findings. However, the full report should contain a detailed description of the methods used in the study. This section is included in order to enable the reader to evaluate the quality of the methods used, to avoid similar mistakes if any were made, and to use similar or identical methods in future projects.

The quality of a research study and its findings is only as good as the validity and reliability of the research methods used to collect data. It is therefore necessary that readers be given the opportunity to make a critical appraisal of the methods by being able to study them in the report. When a part of the research is published and does not include a detailed description of the methods used, in an article for example, the reader must be referred to the complete report in order to provide the opportunity for it to be read and for the quality of the methods used to be judged.

An important function of a literature review as part of every piece of research is to provide an opportunity to learn from the problems experienced and from mistakes made by other researchers. The methods section must therefore discuss all problems encountered and their solutions and the shortcomings and strengths of the methods used.

Another reason for reviewing the literature before undertaking a study is to identify previously used methods which can be used or adapted in the planned study. Unless these are described in considerable detail in the report, readers will be unable to judge their value or otherwise in completed studies.

READERSHIP AND LANGUAGE OF THE REPORT

When writing a report, the needs of its readership are a major consideration as is the need to use a language that readers will understand. Although the formal language may be English, for example, decisions must be made about the use of technical terms, mathematical language and illustrative material such as photographs, tables and figures.

Readership of the report

The report may be written in different ways depending on its intended readership in the knowledge that, for example, a reader with a background in research will have needs which differ from those of the general public most of whom have no such experience.

The general public

Because many readers in the general public may have limited professional or research background and skills, they require a jargon-free and
relatively non-technical report. A report of this type may say very little
about the reviewed literature or research design. Instead emphasis is
placed on presenting, interpreting and discussing the findings.

An examiner

If the report (a dissertation or thesis, for example) is being submitted for
examination, it must comply with the marking and examination criteria
set by the institution concerned. Such a work may focus on the theoretical and philosophical aspects of the research in addition to the more
practical issues.

Dissertations and theses deliberately deal with a number of issues
which are not part of that particular study but an understanding of which
indicates an understanding of the research process generally. For
example, the researcher may discuss a range of *potential* ethical issues
and their possible solutions, although these were not actually experienced. In this way the writer indicates an understanding of an important
aspect of research although it did not actually arise.

A commissioning institution

If the research has been commissioned by an institution or organization,
it is prudent to agree on the probable length and general structure of the
final report as early as possible. It would clearly be problematical if a
50 000-word report in the style and level of a PhD thesis was produced
when the commissioning body hoped for a 10 000-word report which
could be read and understood by a wide readership with limited research
knowledge.

It may be necessary to prepare and circulate a summary to a large
number of people for information or comment. In this instance a
summarized version of the entire work may have to be prepared by
reducing it: 50 000 words to 1000 words would not be uncommon. If
such a summary is required, this needs to be made known in advance as
should its specifications, including length. Although the readership of
the summary will be varied, a limited knowledge of research language
and a general understanding of the subject of the research may be
assumed unless the writer is informed otherwise.

Other researchers

Other researchers may be particularly interested in the research
methods used. Indeed an article extracted from the whole report may

deal only with the research method. Similarly, full details of the statistical analyses, if used, would be included in a report prepared for other researchers. A knowledge of research, technical and statistical language may be assumed of this readership.

Specialists in the subject of the research

Specialists, such as others in the same discipline, may require a report, or report summary, in which the application of the findings to clinical practice is fully discussed. A knowledge of technical language and the subject of the research would be assumed of this readership.

Language of the report

The language of the report is to a large extent dependent on its readership and will include the use of words and possibly mathematical language and pictorial elements in the form of graphs and figures. It is unlikely that the report language will be exclusively of one kind, a combination of two or three types being more common.

Vocabulary

Words must be chosen carefully and written in a clear and understandable way. Reports that are badly written are difficult to read and are frequently not implemented for this reason. Readers are entitled to be critical of a work that is difficult to read. An ambiguous, unclear and otherwise badly written report may reflect muddled thinking by its writer. It is sad that an otherwise good piece of research will have less impact than it deserves because it is badly written.

Mathematical language

Although not all research uses numbers and other mathematical symbols, they form an important, perhaps crucial, part of many studies. They may be used in tables and figures, in the text or to describe statistical concepts or findings. The range and complexity varies from the simple ('Five per cent of the sample was female') to the complex, as used in many statistical tests.

Some health care professionals have difficulty with mathematical language. If it is used in the report for anything other than basic descriptive statistics (percentages and averages, for example), the writer should consider whether some explanation is needed. This decision will obviously depend on the readership, researchers requiring less explanation than professionals with no research background.

Pictorial language (illustrations)

It is a truism that a picture can paint a thousand words. This applies particularly when writing a research report. The types of illustrations used include tables, graphs, line drawings, sociograms, photographs and blueprints. These are sufficiently significant to the subject of writing to justify a chapter being devoted to the subject (see Chapter 8).

GENERAL HINTS FOR WRITING RESEARCH REPORTS

These hints are directed in particular at those writing a report for the first time. The list is not exhaustive, the hallmark of good report writing being innovation, imagination and experimentation with a variety of approaches.

Time

A common error made by beginners is underestimating the time needed to write a report. In general it is prudent to allocate one-third of the time available to the entire project to writing the report. This writing-up time will not necessarily all be used at the end of the time allocated to the research. Perhaps one-half of the writing-up time – one-sixth of the total research time – will be used as the work is proceeding, the other half being used at the end of the project.

Starting to write

Writing the report begins as soon as possible, when ideas about the work first begin to develop. Written work must be produced, however sketchy and disorganized, at every stage of the study. These first draft notes will form an important basis for the final report.

Experience will show that ideas are rarely fully developed and clarified until they are placed on paper. It is easy to be vague and ambiguous in one's thinking, and even in verbal discussions. However, these faults will be more easily identified and rectified when the material is placed on paper.

The writer should state reasons for being interested in this particular research topic and why the research is felt to be necessary; as much background information as possible must be included.

References

All references consulted in relation to the study should be recorded and stored in an alphabetical card or computer system. The record must contain full bibliographical detail of the reference, a summary of its contents, and a note of where it can be found again. If the reference was consulted and found to be of no value to the study, this fact should be noted. *This important aspect of undertaking a research study is initiated as soon as the decision is taken to start the work It is essential to the successful completion of the research report.* (See Chapter 6 for a full description of this subject.)

Documents

All documents relating to the study, those collected as data and those used to collect data, must be clearly labelled and stored for later use. Many will be presented in the body of the report or as appendices. If there is serious doubt as to whether a document needs to be included, it is advisable to err on the side of inclusion.

Structure

A provisional structure of the final report must be drafted during the planning stage of the research. As far as possible this draft should contain as much detail as can be anticipated: chapters/major sections, headings, subheadings, and titles of figures, tables, line drawings and appendices, for example.

The initial draft structure can of course be modified and remodified as the research progresses, with each subsequent draft structure adding considerably to the ease with which the report is written.

Shape

The grouping of material into chapters and sections of chapters, and the sequence of these parts, are what is meant here by 'shape'. The shape of the report both in terms of chapters and their sequence, and in terms of the arrangement of material within chapters, requires careful consideration.

The size of each part of the report and its size as a proportion of the work as a whole must be deliberate rather than left to chance. This decision will be influenced by the purpose of the report and its intended readership.

Title

A tentative title for the report must be decided on at the beginning of the study to provide both a focus for the work and a 'label' by which it becomes known to others. The title is re-examined as the work progresses and can be changed if it fails to encapsulate and accurately reflect the subject of the research. However, it is probable that such a change will be in emphasis only, rather than a completely new title.

Gimmicky titles are best avoided as they often fail to indicate the content of the report to potential readers.

Detail

Good research and well written reports depend greatly on attention to detail. The content of the report must be exact, specific, unambiguous and sufficiently detailed as to leave readers in no doubt about its meaning. Although some professionals regard the detail required of a research report to be pedantic and unnecessary, these are essential features of successful research.

Accuracy

As in all forms of writing, a research report demands a high level of accuracy in the presentation of factual material which has emerged from the research. Although this accuracy is an important feature of the presentation of numerical data, it is by no means confined to that application. Whether qualitative or quantitative data are being described, the material must be checked and rechecked for accuracy. This checking must include the data and research findings and the means used to describe them. An otherwise excellent piece of research must not become 'suspect' because of a lack of attention to accuracy in the report.

Drafts

The writer should allow for making a number of drafts of the report. This will be expensive in time *and* finance if a typist is used, and should be taken into account when budgeting for time and money. In earlier drafts it is important to allow for making changes and additions. This will be made easier if wide margins are left and if paper and pencil are used on one side of the page only. Better still, all drafts can be typed on a word processor which will cope easily with all manner of corrections, changes, additions, moving of text and so on.

Earlier drafts should be shown to and discussed with colleagues or those for whom the work is being prepared. If the research is being formally supervised, all drafts will be read and commented on by supervisors.

The final report should be attractively typed, easy to read, and professionally presented. With minimal effort and relatively little expense, a research report of poor quality in terms of appearance can be transformed into a visually attractive item. This is not to suggest that high quality presentation can ever be a substitute for high quality content. However, poor quality presentation detracts considerably from good content. Readers expect and deserve reports which are carefully prepared.

Summary (abstract)

Whether or not a short summary (abstract) is requested by those for whom the report is being prepared, it is as well to prepare one. Summaries (abstracts) may be 500–1000 words long. It needs considerable skill to write and summarize the entire content of the report. However, this skill will be developed by writing many drafts, by sharing them with colleagues, and by reading successful summaries/abstracts in other reports, particularly those that have been published in article form.

Confidentiality and anonymity

Unless those institutions, groups and individuals who have taken part in the study (by providing data, for example) have agreed to be identified, readers of the report should be unable to identify them. Confidentiality and anonymity can be maintained by stating generally thus:

'A 400-bed district general hospital . . .'
   or
'A sample of patients in a rural location . . .'
   or
'A staff nurse said . . .'
   or
'A consultant physician reported that . . .'

PUBLISHING RESEARCH REPORTS

Research reports may be published in the form of the written word or by other means such as papers read at conferences or study days. It is necessary that the report be made available to those who commissioned the research, and possibly, in either complete or summary form, to those who participated in it. This is particularly the case where data have been collected from fellow professionals. Unless there has been any prior agreement to restrict circulation of the report, an effort should be made to make it available to as wide an appropriate readership as possible. This is often most effectively achieved by publishing a series of articles or by converting the report into 'book form' for publication.

In summary, the preparation of a research report involves a number of steps in addition to those required for other types of writing for a professional readership. Although the writer has the advantage of working from a pre-existing blueprint in the form of the structure of the research process and of the selected research design, the accuracy, detail and objectivity required in writing a research report call for careful attention, as is the case in all good writing.

Chapters 14
Dissertations and Theses

A thesis, plural theses, is the term given to research-based written work produced as a requirement for higher degree studies such as Doctor of Philosophy or Master of Philosophy. In many countries, including the United Kingdom, dissertations are often a requirement for courses other than those leading to a higher degree. For example, students on a degree or diploma course at a university or college of higher education, or those undertaking some Master of Science courses, may have to produce a dissertation. The work is prepared under the close supervision of an appropriate staff member of the institution to which it will be submitted, and of an external supervisor in some instances.

The differences in required writing skills between dissertations and theses are sufficiently small as to make a combined discussion of them appropriate. All the points made in this discussion apply equally to dissertations and theses, although some dissertations may be more limited in their depth and scope than some theses. In the interests of brevity, only the word 'dissertation' will be used; however, the word should be interpreted as meaning dissertations *and* theses.

As far as possible all materials collected and written in connection with a dissertation must be duplicated and the 'extra' copy kept separate from the original. This is to safeguard against the unlikely, although possible, loss of the only copy of the work. As is the case with any written material, including that submitted to a publisher, the writer should consider using registered mail or recorded delivery if it is to be mailed.

STRUCTURE

The structure and subsequent appearance of a dissertation are particularly important. Structural requirements vary between institutions and occasionally between teachers and supervisors; Examples 35 and 36 are typical. It is important to ensure that the specific requirements of the institution for which the work is being prepared are obtained and adhered to.

The dissertation consists of three major parts: those items that precede the actual dissertation, the dissertation material, and finally those items that follow it. It is traditional to number the pages that precede the dissertation proper in Roman numerals. The pages of the dissertation, starting with the first page of the first chapter, should be numbered in Arabic numerals. Items that come after the body of the dissertation should be numbered consecutively with the dissertation itself. Although details on arrangement may vary, Example 35 is typical: it shows the title page, the first typewritten page inside the binding (page i).

Example 35

Title page of dissertation

Title of the work, for example:

Professional Relationships in Health care

Name and qualifications

Submitted in partial fulfilment of the degree of [title of degree or diploma] of [name of the institution awarding the degree or diploma]

Title of the degree or diploma

Name of the institution or degree-awarding body

Year of submission

The next page should be a 'contents page'. This should be an exact reflection of the dissertation and should contain every major item in it. Example 36 is one type of dissertation structure.

Example 36

Sample dissertation structure

Contents

Page number

Once the contents, and therefore the structure of the work, have been described, each item in the contents page follows in the sequence shown.

- *List of tables.* The list of tables should include the number and full title of each table and the page number on which it appears. The order of the listed tables should be as they appear in the text, Table 1 appearing first, Table 2 second and so on.
- *List of figures.* The list of figures is similar to the list of tables, with the figures within the text listed by number, for example Figure 1, title and page number.
- *List of appendices.* The number or letter (for example Appendix 1 or Appendix A), title and page number of each appendix, which will be located at the end of the dissertation, should appear here.
- *Acknowledgements.* The help of those individuals, institutions or groups which have made completion of the dissertation possible should be acknowledged here.
- *Summary.* The inclusion of a summary of the entire work, written to a specific and predetermined length, is a frequent requirement in dissertations. The word 'abstract' is sometimes used instead of 'summary', depending on the institution.

Each of the preceding five items should begin on a new page and must be well presented in terms of structure and given maximum visual appeal by the use of good layout and typing skills.

- *Chapters.* The chapters or major sections of the dissertation must now appear. Each must begin on a new page and be given a number such as 'Chapter 1' and an appropriately descriptive title.
- *Appendices.* Each appendix must also begin on a new page and have a unique letter or number such as 'Appendix 1' or 'Appendix A' and an appropriately descriptive title.
- *Reference list.* All references cited in the text, either by para-phrasing or by direct quotation, must now be listed under the title 'Reference list' or 'References'. The form in which the references are presented will depend on the reference system used in the text: the Harvard or numerical system, for example. See Chapter 5 for a full discussion of reference use and presentation.
- *Bibliography.* A bibliography containing those references that relate to the subject of the dissertation and that were consulted

during its preparation should be included if it is felt that this will be of value to the reader.

BINDING

Dissertations invariably have to be bound to meet the very specific requirements of the institution for which it is being prepared. Binding facilities may be available within the institution or may have to be arranged with a commercial binder. In either event it is essential that the precise requirements, in terms of size, colour, style and form of binding, be made known to those undertaking the binding.

INFORMATION FOR THE TYPIST

In all but a very few instances, dissertations are submitted in typescript format. The reasons for this requirement include the following.

First, the use of typescript ensures that the reader can understand the material. Although some handwriting is relatively easy to read, it is often tiring or difficult to read for a long period.

Secondly, if dissertations are to be made for public or general use, through inter-library loans for example, they must be presented in professionally prepared typescript.

Thirdly, there is no doubt that a reader, and possibly an examiner, will be positively influenced by material which is attractively typed and professionally presented. This is also of particular importance when submitting material for publication. It is not being suggested that a good visual presentation is a substitute for poor content, but busy readers do prefer material that has optimum visual appeal.

Finally, the typewriter, or more commonly the word processor, is much more accurate, versatile and consistent than the human hand, producing a much better quality of work. Whenever possible, the technology of the typewriter or, increasingly, the word processor should be fully exploited for the final draft. See Chapter 21 (Writing Technology) for a discussion of the advantages and scope of word processor use.

The following discussion contains selected specifications which are made available to a typist. It is not exhaustive: a good typist will almost certainly raise further specific points requiring clarification.

Completion date

A realistic completion date for the work, with some time for emergencies, must be discussed and agreed with the typist. Both writer and typist may benefit from setting completion dates for each major part of the dissertation. A typist will need adequate time to work on the dissertation, particularly if he or she is doing the work in addition to another job. The items considered in working to a timetable and completion date are:

Date/time for each of various drafts (including discussion with supervisor/s)
Date/time for preparing penultimate draft (including discussion with supervisor/s)
Date/time for proofreading penultimate draft
Date/time for typing final draft
Time required for professional binding
Submission of dissertation

Paper size and typing style

Typing paper comes in a variety of shapes and sizes. Although A4 (210 mm × 297 mm) is the most commonly used paper size in the United Kingdom, there are a number of other sizes some of which are more popular in other countries. If you are not supplying the typist with paper, ensure that clear instructions about paper size are given.

Style relates to such items as the line spacing to be used, margin size, numbering of pages and the reference system used. Spacing may be single, $1\frac{1}{2}$ or double; the lower the spacing number, single spacing for example, the greater will be the number of lines of typescript on the page.

Margin size instructions may range from 'an appropriate margin size' to an exact margin requirement in relation to all four margins. For example the margins of a dissertation may have to be:

Lower margin: 40 mm
Upper margin: 20 mm
Left margin: 20 mm
Right margin: 10 mm

Page numbering specifications may relate to the exact position of the page number: in the centre of the lower margin 10 mm from the lower edge, for example. Roman numerals might be requested in the preliminary parts of the work, Arabic numerals being used in the main text. It might be prudent to ask the typist to number the pages lightly in pencil and refrain from typing the numbers until the final draft stage is reached. Thus if material has to be removed or added, it will not be necessary to change all page numbers.

The reference system should be carefully explained in order that the typist can keep a check on its use by the writer.

Quality of paper

The quality of paper to be used, usually described in weight, may be specified. If no such specification is made, it is best to use a high quality paper.

Italicizing and underlining

Handwritten work may contain some sections or individual words to be underlined or italicized in the final typewritten dissertation. Although all typewriters will have an underlining facility, some may not be able to italicize. Virtually all word processors will be able to do both.

Provided that clear instructions are given to the typist, these stylistic variations will present no difficulty. For example, the instruction might be given that 'Items underlined in blue/black ink should remain underlined, and items underlined in red ink should be italicized'.

Inserting extra pages

If additional pages are inserted into a completed dissertation, the page numbers of the original text need not be changed if they have already been typed in. Rather, the additional pages can be added with letters after the page number. Thus, two pages inserted after page 9 would be marked 9a and 9b.

Headings

Even the most unsophisticated typewriter will cope with at least three orders of headings, which are typed without underlining and without a full stop at the end. As headings appear in the handwritten work, their rank must be indicated in the margin by placing an encircled 1 to the left of the most important heading, 2 to the left of the next, most important, and 3 to the left of the heading of least importance (where there are only three heading grades). The typist should be informed that major headings 1 are to be capitalized and centred, that subheadings 2 are to be centred with only the first letter of main words capitalized, and that sub-subheadings 3 are to begin at the left margin and that only the first letter of the first word and all proper nouns are to be capitalized. Thus the three levels of heading must appear in the handwritten work as:

① REHABILITATION OF THE ELDERLY
② Aspects of Multidisciplinary Teamwork
③ Rehabilitative occupational therapy

The inclusion of the numbers, which are omitted from the typescript, will ensure that the typist will be in no doubt as to the heading rank.

OTHER SPECIFICATIONS

The specifications of the body, examiner or institution for which the dissertation is being prepared should be obtained and studied. The nature and amount of specification detail provided varies considerably between institutions. Details of the following are often provided.

Abbreviations

Over-reliance on abbreviations should be avoided. Once a term has been stated in full *and* abbreviated in the text (National Health Service (NHS) for example), the abbreviated form should be used subsequently. Those that should be avoided are etc., i.e. and e.g. as they are easily overused when little attempt is made to find alternatives.

Quotation marks

Quotation marks (inverted commas) are used mostly to identify passages that have been quoted from other people's work. They may also be placed around words used in an unusual context or coined for a specific purpose. In the UK it is usual to use single inverted commas for quotations, and double ones for words quoted within quotations. In the US the opposite applies.

Number of copies

It is usual to make a copy or copies for the person to whom the dissertation is to be submitted and one further copy for the author. Clearly, the required number must be established *before* binding takes place. When two or more copies are required, as is invariably the case, there are two ways of doing this. First, if the typing has been done on a word processor, then multiple copies can be produced. Secondly, the original typed dissertation, whether produced on a typewriter or on a word processor, can be photocopied. The number of institutions and individuals that do not accept photocopies is small and decreasing, and it is the case that contemporary copying machines make copies which are every bit as good as the original.

SUPERVISION

All aspects of writing, including the planning phase, must be discussed fully with the dissertation supervisor. It is standard practice to submit handwritten work, particularly in its earlier drafts, to the supervisor, who will examine it thoroughly, make comment and give advice.

Chapter 15
Articles

Articles form a key part of the professional literature, offering ideal opportunities for the novice and the experienced writer, those who have a short sharp message to convey, and those who want to say something of relatively immediate significance. The existence of so many journals that serve the health professions testifies to the importance of the article as a means of professional communication.

An unfortunate myth surrounds the writing of articles for publication. It is often perceived as something which an unspecified 'they' do, and which is beyond the scope of most professionals. The reality is that publishing in the form of articles is the business of *every* health care professional, and that 'they' neither deserve nor wish to have a monopoly on this activity.

Journal editors are constantly on the lookout for new ideas and fresh material. Contrary to popular belief they are more than willing to consider and accept manuscripts from those trying to publish for the first time. Provided that due attention is given to preparation, structure and content, most professionally written manuscripts will be published. The number of journals that can be approached is large, since it includes those from all the countries that publish in the writer's native language. Indeed those who speak a second language or have access to a translator should seriously consider publishing in a language other than their own.

In identifying a subject about which to write, the aspiring author should select the one with which they are most familiar. There are topics of which anyone in the health care field has a unique experience and knowledge and is therefore qualified to write about. Many professionals perceive their work as 'routine', 'basic' and 'ordinary' and assume that others could not possibly be interested in reading an account of it. The reality is that every aspect of health care has the potential to become the subject of a journal article; it simply requires sufficient imagination and innovativeness to identify features of it that will be of interest to readers. It is not being suggested that any description of any activity or idea should be prepared for publication, particularly if this has been done many times before. Rather, the subject of the publication is no more important than the ability of the writer to look at it in a new way, to increase knowledge of it, to develop new relationships between known facts, and to challenge existing beliefs regarding established treatments or procedures.

The major steps in having an article published are planning, writing and publishing. These will be dealt with in turn, as will each of their parts.

PLANNING

Planning begins with a commitment to writing for publication generally, and to writing an article in particular. At this stage the intending writer must decide whether to produce the article personally, or involve a colleague, who may or may not have publishing experience as a co-author. This decision, a matter of personal preference, has advantages and disadvantages.

Co-authorship

A contribution from one or more co-authors should be considered only if it is known that the article needs this type of authorship, and that the others are willing and able to play a *full* part in its construction. Some papers, even relatively short ones, have as many as seven or more authors, and such a large number is usually hard to justify. Some may have been included because they happen to be in charge of the unit in which the principal author works, because they are a senior colleague, or simply because they expect to be included. A basic rule is that the number of authors should be kept to a minimum, and that only those who make a significant contribution to the paper should be listed as co-authors. The writer should beware of literary hitchhikers who expect credit for work they have not done.

Whether co-authors are senior or junior colleagues, from the same or another discipline, and experienced or inexperienced writers, will vary according to the needs of the paper and its senior author. If more than one author is involved, unambiguous decisions must be made regarding division of responsibilities, how costs should be met, and how income if any should be distributed.

If one or more co-authors are involved, clear arrangements must be made concerning who will be the principal (first-named) author, and the sequence of the names of the remainder if there is more than one co-author. It is *not* the case that the names of the authors of a multiauthor paper should necessarily be listed in alphabetical order, except in the highly unlikely event of there being no principal author or that all co-authors have made an equal contribution. In that case it might be as well to decide the order of names by drawing them out of a hat, despite protestations from contributor A.A. Aarhus! In general, the first-named author is regarded as the principal author of the work and the co-authors as having a supporting role. The person who initiates the article idea, contacts potential co-authors, produces the first written material, provides the momentum for the work, and puts the final product together is given senior author status and is first named in the list of authors.

The idea

With a little effort a number of ideas which could usefully form the basis of an article can be identified. However, the motivation to publish must be equalled by a conviction that the information needs to be shared with professional colleagues. Specific reasons for writing include informing, educating, speculating, questioning, identifying issues, influencing opinion, and enhancing career prospects. These reasons were outlined in Chapter 1 and need no further discussion here.

As the subject of the article emerges, the writer must ask the following questions to determine its suitability. If the answer to each question is 'Yes', then the chances of successfully producing and publishing an article are very good.

Am I sufficiently interested in the subject? Although writing for publication is a rewarding experience, it can be difficult. Unless there is a keen interest in, and commitment to, the subject of the writing, the level of motivation will not be high enough to sustain writing through the difficult periods.

Do I have the necessary experience, knowledge and understanding of the subject? The subject of the article must be one of which the writer has an intimate knowledge. In most instances writers choose a subject that has formed a significant part of their work experience. In the unlikely event of attraction to a subject which, although of considerable interest, is outside immediate experience, it is important to take time to research the topic to become sufficiently well versed in it. Although it *might* be possible to convince an editor that one has a greater knowledge of a subject than is actually the case, this deficiency will quickly be spotted by unforgiving readers of the article, as can be seen in the 'Letters to the Editor' pages of many professional journals.

Is the subject of the article novel, newsworthy, or presented in a new way? Although there is some merit in re-examining old ideas and reinforcing established practice, editors are justifiably more interested in original ideas and those that advance professional knowledge. To be able to answer this question positively, a potential author must have researched the subject very thoroughly.

Is the information accurate and factual? Any information which is presented as fact must be thoroughly checked and rechecked. Anything presented as opinion must be clearly differentiated from that presented as fact. A common error made by many beginners is to confuse fact with opinion. So far as is possible, readers should be able to check on factual material. However, if they are unable to do so, they will be obliged to rely on the ability of the writer to present it correctly.

Is the material important enough to share with professional colleagues? The relevance of the material to professional practice, management, research or education should be clear. Although there is some room in professional journals for papers that have a distinct theoretical basis, those with a clear practical application are valued by readers and editors.

Few writers are able to produce publishable ideas on demand. It may be useful to keep a small file of ideas as they occur, making a note of why they seemed important at the time. Flashes of inspiration will only become pearls of wisdom if they can be recalled at a later stage.

Where to publish

A large number of journals serve the health care professions. Some are highly specialized, many have a more general readership. Some are specific to one discipline, others are multidisciplinary. In order to decide where to publish, the range of possible options should be discussed with a specialist librarian. A good professional library will have copies of most relevant journals and will be able to obtain back copies of those not in stock.

If the article is highly specialized, it will be necessary to choose journals that either deal with that specialty or that have a broad readership. There would be little point in submitting an article about post-mastectomy care to a journal specializing in infectious diseases. Conversely, almost any article, provided that it is not too specialized, might be submitted to a journal with a general readership.

Guides to contributors

Once a shortlist of perhaps three to five journals has been identified as being suitable, the guides which their publishers produce for contributors must be obtained and studied. Contributors' guides will be found inside every issue of some journals and inside some issues of others, or can be obtained by writing to the editors of yet others.

The quality of information which these guides contain varies considerably between journals. Typically they give details of typing requirements, number of copies, length, reference system to be used, and the types of illustration that are suitable. If, even after obtaining a guide to contributors, there are any doubts as to the possible requirements of a journal, further specific questions can be directed to the editor.

In addition the articles that appear in the shortlisted journals should be examined closely in order to get a feel for the type, quality and range of material that has been acceptable to that publication. Having considered the content and requirements of a few selected journals, a firm decision must then be made about the choice of journal. The article is now being prepared with a specific journal in mind, rather than having to find a journal to suit the article.

ARTICLE STRUCTURE

Next, the idea must be developed into a draft structure. The first task is to decide on a title. Although the title is tentative and may well change as the work progresses, it does serve to give an important focus for, and direction to, the article.

The first draft of the major headings to be used is now written down and is produced by 'thinking around' the subject of the paper. At this stage there is no need to be over-concerned about the order of the ideas: the writer should just jot them down. The major headings can be then rearranged and have the subheadings and sub-subheadings added in the same way. Although this structure will be modified as the article progresses, it is a logical starting point from which to work. The major and subsidiary parts of the article should be neither too few nor too many. Too many result in a disjointed and difficult to read paper, too few and overlong sections may be equally difficult and tedious to read. In case of doubt it may be useful to read some published papers to get a feel for this aspect of structure.

Example 37 demonstrates how a typical structure might look after a number of drafts.

Finding a publisher

The next task is to find a journal editor who will be willing to give an 'in principle' indication of serious interest in the article. This arrangement will, of course, depend on the acceptability of the final manuscript. However, it gives a fairly firm indication of interest on the part of the editor. If, from the shortlist of appropriate journals, it is found that there is more than one journal that would be suitable, the convention is to get in touch with one journal at a time.

Finding a potential publisher is done by submitting the article structure along with a query letter. (See Example 38.) The letter is short and to the point, asking for no more than an expression of interest on the part of the editor. It should be borne in mind that an editor cannot accept a manuscript until it has been submitted in its entirety. The editor's response to the query letter and the enclosed outline may be one of three: first, a definite expression of interest, in which case writing the article should proceed; secondly, interest in publishing if certain specified changes are made, in which case the writer should proceed to meet the editor's requirements; thirdly, the editor may reject the proposal

Example 37

Sample structure of content of article

The development of health care research

Introduction (overview/summary of paper)
The nature and purpose of health care research
  The nature of research
    Research principles
    Universality of health care research
  The purpose of health care research
    To advance health care knowledge
    To re-examine current clinical practice
    To identify further research questions
The development of health care research
  Development nationally
  Areas of individual development
  Areas of institutional development
Future developments
  Government-sponsored research
    Research fellowships
    Funding of research units
  Privately funded research
    Self-supporting research
    Privately commissioned research
Conclusions and discussion

because it 'does not meet with present requirements', in which case another journal should be tried. Now that the planning phase is complete, work on preparing the full manuscript begins.

Not all writers submit an article summary and query letter to editors; many submit the completed article with a covering letter. Either approach is acceptable and depends on the personal preference of the author.

WRITING THE ARTICLE

At this stage, getting the words on paper is far more important than achieving an excellent writing style. Many beginners have difficulty because they (wrongly) believe that there is an 'ideal' writing style to which they should conform. Provided that it is clear and readable, a personal writing style should be used. There is no universally correct recipe for success in writing the article, but the following guidelines may be useful.

Research the subject

In this context the word *research* relates to finding out as much as possible about the subject by reading about it and discussing it with

Example 38 _____

Query letter

Ward 2
Medical Unit
General Hospital
Finsbury Street
Norman ED3 13H
England
Date

Ms M Bryant
Editor
Journal of Health Care Research
1 Farlane Avenue
Risseville
New Jersey 2415
USA

Dear Ms Bryant,

The Development of Health Care Research

I write to enquire if *Journal of Health Care Research* would be interested in the above manuscript which I am currently preparing. The paper examines the general development of health care research and speculates about the future direction of this development (see enclosed structure and contents).

The manuscript, which will comply with the editorial requirements of your journal, will be ready for submission approximately 3 months from this date.

I look forward to hearing from you and hope you are able to give this proposal your favourable consideration. I shall, of course, be delighted to receive any comments or suggestions you may have regarding the enclosed outline.

Yours sincerely,

Name, qualifications, position.

_____

colleagues. Although the subject will be chosen because it is of special interest and of relevance to the writer's professional life, there is almost certainly much more information available about it than is realized. By researching the subject, therefore, the writer will be better able to produce an informative, insightful and well informed article that will be more satisfying to readers. Discussing the subject with colleagues plays an important part in all phases of writing.

Obtaining permission (if needed)

When the contents of the article relate to any identifiable person or institution, permission for the material to be published must be obtained. One way of avoiding this issue is to refer to persons as Miss X or Mr Z, or to refer to an institution as 'a district general hospital', for example. Great care must be taken with anonymity. If this cannot be achieved, permission must be obtained.

If any of the ideas or materials referred to (a new clinical technique, for example) have been developed in the writer's place of work, then the permission of the employer must be obtained. When permission of any kind is being asked, the general content of the article must be made known and the specific information relating to the individual or institution must also be made available. Ideally, permission should be obtained in writing; verbal permission is sensibly followed by a letter acknowledging with thanks the details of the permission granted.

In those instances when permission need not be obtained (where the article makes no reference to a place of work and does not identify specific individuals or institutions), it may be decided to inform others of the intention to publish. For example, it might be prudent to inform clinical or managerial colleagues. Once the article is accepted for publication it might be as well, particularly if working within an organizational structure, to send a copy to colleagues 'for information'.

Developing the structure

The previously prepared structure must now be developed further by being examined, rearranged and altered as necessary and extended by the addition of one or more sentences to each of its parts. It is at this stage that writing blocks may be experienced. The following hints are intended to minimize these.

- An environment that is conducive to writing must be found. This varies from person to person and can only be found by experimenting. For some it is the lounge in front of the television set; for others their bedroom or the college or public library.
- The writer must get their thoughts on paper, irrespective of how disorganized they appear. It is important to remember that perfection may never be achieved, and certainly not in the first draft. Subsequent drafts can be used to rearrange, improve and extend the material.
- The writer should always use pieces of paper of the same size, should write (in pencil if practical) or type on one side of the paper, and should always leave large margins around the edges of the paper and in between various sections of the manuscript. This will enable

'cutting and pasting' and rearranging work in the next draft. The use of a word processor should be seriously considered.

- When writing, ideas relating to both earlier and later parts of the paper will emerge. The writer should not be tempted to go back to the earlier part of the paper, or to commence work on the later stages. However, any ideas emerging at this stage must be noted in writing for use later or when writing a subsequent draft.
- It is important to think about how the quality of the manuscript might be improved by the use of graphic presentations, that is, the use of anything other than words. The proposed positions of such illustrations should be noted; their form and content can be worked out in detail at a later stage.
- The writer should never regard what has been written as unchangeable. Subsequent editing will improve the manuscript.
- Some time should be allowed to elapse between each draft. A few days may be necessary to enable additional ideas to develop and mature. Trusted colleagues who are familiar with the subject area should be asked to read and comment on each draft.
- It is important to make full use of a thesaurus, a dictionary and other reference texts.

Article content

In large part the previously constructed structure of the article will determine its content. Thus, if the structure has been well planned, making decisions about the content will be easy.

The writer should think of the article in terms of three major parts contained within the overall structure. They are: the introduction, the body and the conclusion.

Introduction (around 15% of total length)

The introduction is undoubtedly the 'shop window' of the manuscript as not only is it the first part to be seen but also it plays a large part in making potential readers decide whether or not to read the rest of the paper. The first few sentences of the introduction should capture readers' attention and persuade them to read the remainder. It should set the tone for the rest of the paper and must include a brief outline of its contents.

Body of the paper (around 70% of total length)

The main body of the paper is the longest and most important part, and might be the most difficult to write. During this phase of writing, it is important to refer frequently to the previously prepared structure.

Indeed, the body of the article emerges from an expansion and elaboration of the structure.

The major challenges likely to be met at this stage relate to decisions concerning the amount of detail required; ensuring that the paper has a logical sequence; holding the interest of the reader; and maintaining a fluent writing style. Meeting these challenges is a matter of personal judgement, and very few hard and fast rules apply. It is important to be critical of the work and to encourage colleagues to whom the draft copies are shown to be likewise.

Conclusion and discussion (around 15% of total length)

The principal functions of the third section are to draw the article to a close, to make a concluding statement, to summarize the major features of the paper, and to give direction to the possible development of the issues raised. As with all other parts of the paper, the concluding section must be carefully planned, written and rewritten.

Further drafts

The process described in the preceding paragraphs must be repeated over and over again until the manuscript has been satisfactorily completed. Although the perfect manuscript has never been written, the aspiring author will want to do as well as possible. In deciding how many drafts to write there comes a point at which the law of diminishing returns applies, when only minimal improvement can be gained from writing yet another draft. It is now time to show the paper to a colleague for final comment before it is submitted prior to yet another thorough presubmission check.

Presubmission check

- *Grammar, structure, headings, subheadings, page numbers and length* must be checked. The article must be clear, readable and fluently written. All the requirements of the publisher must be met, and any necessary deviations such as reasonable additional length must be made known to the editor.
- *Accuracy, content and presentation of all tables and figures* must be checked. Illustration titles must describe the content of each presentation, be referred to in the text close to where they are to appear, and be constructed to give maximum impact.
- The *title* must be checked to make sure it really describes the content of the article; all other headings, subheadings and sub-subheadings must be checked too.
- *Sequence and length* of all parts of the paper must be checked.
- All *references* must be checked and rechecked. Questions to ask

when checking references include: do all those cited in the text appear in the reference list?; and does the reference system used conform to the journal's requirements, and is it used correctly and consistently throughout? All quotations in the text must now be compared with the publications in which they originated, and must be identical. All items in the reference list must be examined and compared with the original documents or with carefully prepared notes taken from them. The names of the authors, years of publication, titles of publications and all other bibliographical data must be checked and rechecked.

- It is necessary to check that appropriate *permission to publish* has, if necessary, been obtained, and that this has been confirmed in writing. A copy of the paper should be sent to colleagues for information.
- Any additional material that is to be enclosed, other than the actual article, must be checked. Examples include acknowledgement of assistance and/or permission, name (or names) and details of co-author/s if any, and photographs and other items.
- The content and structure of the covering letter that will be enclosed with the article must be checked. Such a letter will, of course, be unique, and its content will be influenced by whether or not there has been previous correspondence such as a query letter. Example 39 shows a typical covering letter and illustrates some of the points that might usefully included.

PUBLISHING

If an acknowledgement of receipt of the manuscript has not been received by the end of two weeks (although it is reasonable to expect it by return mail), the writer should get in touch with the editor by phone or another letter and ask if it has arrived. If an affirmative reply is obtained as a result of a phone call, it is important to ensure that this is confirmed in writing.

Acceptance or rejection

It is common for manuscripts to be accepted with suggestions being made for minor or substantial alterations. Beginning writers should pay particular attention to this fact as many are disheartened by what they (wrongly) see as a rejection. However, if the paper is accepted unconditionally, then all that is needed is that the editor be sent a thank you note.

Perhaps the most common form of acceptance is the one in which the writer is asked to make specific changes in the manuscript before resubmission. If these changes are made to meet the editor's require-

Example 39

Covering letter

Ward 2
Medical Unit
General Hospital
Finsbury Street
Norman ED3 13H
England
Date

Ms M. Bryant
Editor
Journal of Health Care Research
1 Farlane Avenue
Risseville
New Jersey 2415
USA

Dear Ms Bryant

The Development of Health Care Research

In response to your letter of [date] in which you expressed an interest in the above manuscript, I enclose two copies which have been prepared to meet the requirements of your journal.

In order that the manuscript can be considered in the context of my professional background, I enclose a copy of my curriculum vitae.

I look forward to your reply and hope you will give the manuscript favourable consideration. As requested in your guide to contributors, I have not submitted the paper to any other journal at present.

Yours sincerely,

Name, qualifications and position

---

ments, there is a good chance that the resubmitted paper will be accepted. Such a request for modification may come from the editor personally, or from one of the editorial staff of the journal.

The length of time between the acceptance and eventual publication of an article varies considerably between journals. It is unlikely to be published in less than 6 months, and it might take up to a year. Although some journals are willing to indicate the approximate time between acceptance and publication, most are only willing to say that the article has been accepted.

In the event of an editor rejecting a manuscript which has been submitted for the first time, the temptation to throw it away or to write an angry letter to the editor must be resisted. Rejection may come in one of two forms and will in either case have something to teach the writer. First, the editor may simply refuse to accept the article and include no further comment. Frustrating although this is, it is a fact of life and one which possibly reflects the large number of manuscripts that reach the editor's desk. In this case the writer should begin to modify the article, if it seems as though that would help, for resubmission to another journal.

Secondly, the editor may give a reason for rejection, for example that 'It does not meet with our present requirements'. Other reasons may be more specific and point to deficiencies in the paper. These reasons must be studied closely and, if possible, used to improve the article which might be resubmitted to the same journal or, as is more often the case, modified for submission to another.

Rejection slips are not the end of the road for a particular manuscript. Their contents should be studied carefully and learned from. If the manuscript has reached this stage of development, there is an extremely good chance that it will be published if the writer perseveres.

WRITER–EDITOR RELATIONSHIP

Contrary to what some potential writers believe, editors are friendly people who try hard to enable and encourage professionals to develop their writing skills to the full. They have an obvious vested interest in stimulating the flow of high quality written material. It would not be in their interest to turn down good manuscripts out of hand or to discourage writers with potential. In order to develop a positive writer–editor relationship, the following points should be borne in mind. The development of mutual trust is essential, requiring both parties to be frank and honest with each other. Writers should expect editors to be totally honest in their opinion about submitted manuscripts, and their critical views should be accepted objectively and professionally rather than interpreted as a personal attack.

Every effort should be made to keep to agreements made in relation to manuscript length or delivery date, for example.

It is best to write to the general editor of the journal, or possibly to the specialist editor, by name. This information can usually be found on or near the contents page in a current copy of the journal. The same article must *never* be submitted to more than one journal simultaneously. Building up a positive working relationship with a journal editor can be a rewarding experience. The fruits of this mutually advantageous personal relationship are undoubtedly better quality manuscripts and increasing publishing opportunities.

Editorial suggestions

Having accepted the manuscript the editor will subject it to the editing process. All articles are professionally edited and, if necessary, considerably improved by editorial input. The job of the editor is to enhance the work whilst maintaining the writer's general writing style, meaning and intention.

The edited manuscript in the form of proofs will be returned for proofreading. The author has the responsibility to make sure that the proofs contain what he or she wants them to contain. The checked work, and any corrections, must be returned to the editor. If the writer feels unhappy about any if the editing, this must be made known to the editor. Because the editor will be working to firm publishing deadlines the proofs must be returned by the agreed dates; three weeks from receipt is not unusual. If the writer expects to be away for more than two weeks from the address to which the proofs will be sent, he or she should inform the editor.

AFTER PUBLICATION

When the article is published, those who read it are entitled, indeed expected, to comment on it. Such comments may take the form of personal correspondence with the writer, letters to the journal in which the article was published, or references to it in subsequent publications. These comments can take the form of criticism, congratulations or discussion of its strengths and weaknesses. The author should accept positive comment graciously, learn from critical comment, and be slightly concerned about the total absence of any comment whatever.

Chapter 16
Curriculum Vitae and Résumé

A curriculum vitae (CV) contains personal biographical information and professional details including training, qualifications, experience, continuing education and other relevant activities such as publications. Apart from personal details such as name and age, entries should start at the point at which the subject became a student in a profession. When opportunities to develop a career are taken, the CV must reflect that development; if an opportunity is lost, the CV will be the poorer for it.

This personal record, which might be used along with an application form for a job, research grant or travel scholarship for example, is a 'shop window' of professional achievements. Relatively inexperienced staff might feel that it is only appropriate to those with more rather than less experience. The fact is that professionals of all levels of experience require a CV from the point of entry as a student. The only difference between the novice and the expert is the nature and volume of the content.

During the past few years commercial companies have been set up to meet the demand for professionally prepared CVs. Individuals supply biographical and professional details and the company provides a well structured and professionally presented CV – at a price of course. Expenditure on such a service may be money wisely spent. Alternatively, with the assistance of an able typist and some knowledge of how to construct a CV, there is considerable advantage in doing the job oneself, particularly if there is access to a word processor. Personal CV writing, with the help of a typist or personal use of a word processor, means that it can be updated and/or adapted for different uses as often as necessary, something which is more expensive if a commercial company is used. If a word processor is used, it is important to retain the disk for updating.

As important as the ability to write a CV is, an understanding of what it represents and how to record a well balanced statement of achievements is also necessary. The resulting document is an accurate account of professional experiences and successes, and must neither understate nor overstate.

Misplaced humility might make some individuals believe that people who write a curriculum vitae do so only to make themselves appear unnecessarily impressive to others. This is, in part, correct. People do produce them to make themselves look good and to impress others; and are perfectly justified both personally and professionally in doing so. Rather than being a considered option, this form of writing is a professional necessity for everyone.

CURRICULUM VITAE OR RÉSUMÉ?

Although the two terms are frequently used interchangeably, their meanings differ in that the résumé is a *summary* of a curriculum vitae. This chapter focuses mainly on the construction of the latter. It concludes by discussing how the CV can be summarized to enable the compilation of a résumé.

CURRICULUM VITAE

Recording entries

All relevant professional activities must be recorded in writing as soon as possible after they occur. This will reduce the need to gather information some time after the event. Unless this is done, entries might be omitted because details are not available or have been forgotten. Thus it is important to note the nature and length of clinical experiences during training; the structure and general content of the syllabus; professional visits; the title and subject of clinical and/or research project involvement; contributions to conferences and study days; and participation in the work of professional organizations. Details of membership of libraries, membership of specialist societies, and the content of all continuing education courses (however short) should also be included.

Early in a career, some of the collected material may seem rather trivial, for example membership of two local professional libraries, or the publication of a short letter in the professional press. The reality is that someone reading the CV of an inexperienced professional will be very interested in such information, which will be useful when comparing applicants who have applied for the same job or travel scholarship, for example. In short, these apparently trivial items are important to anyone who is reading a CV. If in doubt, a record of all potentially important items should still be kept. When compiling the professional record, the writer can then decide whether or not each item is relevant. One of the advantages of preparing it personally, particularly on a word processor, is that it can be adapted and changed in emphasis to suit different occasions. For example, it is likely that a CV that is supporting a job application will emphasize different items from those in a CV used to support an application for a research grant. Similarly, it might be decided to emphasize research, managerial, teaching or clinical attributes, or more than one of these.

As a career develops, the content will include less detail of earlier achievements and focus on more recent ones. For example, whilst detail of initial clinical experiences may be entered in a first CV after qualifying, this will be replaced by detail of subsequent experiences and activities in due course. The content is therefore dynamic and requires updating as a career progresses. Length depends on whether one is a beginner, in mid-career, or nearing the end of a career. More importantly, it depends on the extent to which professional opportunities which deserve inclusion have been both grasped and undertaken successfully. Whereas a novice in any of the professions might have a short CV, a mid-career or senior professional should have a considerably longer record of *relevant* entries. Experienced professionals who do not have a well developed CV that includes a proportion of relevant, substantive and recent entries might reasonably be regarded as professionally less active than a contemporary who has a well developed one. This point will not be lost on an interview panel.

WHEN IS A CV NEEDED?

A curriculum vitae is prepared to enable another person or organization to make a judgement regarding the individual's professional background, achievements and competence. It may be the initial means by which an applicant is judged, and occasionally the only one. Alternatively, it might be accompanied by other information such as an application form or references. Examples of when a CV is needed include:

- Supporting an application for a job, usually, but not always, in addition to an application form and references. It is probably worth while including a CV whether or not one is asked for. It is essential that referees be sent a copy of the CV as soon as they have agreed to provide references. It will help them to construct the reference and will prevent a fallible memory contradicting an important entry.
- As additional material to support a course application.
- As background information for a travel scholarship application.
- As an integral part of an application for research funding, and as a possible appendix to a research proposal.
- To support a higher degree application.
- To support an application to a professional journal from a potential book or manuscript reviewer.
- To meet the needs of those employers who are required to inform one or more organizations of employees' professional achievements, background and so on.
- When being considered as an external examiner to an academic course.

- To convince a publisher that a potential book author or editor has a suitable professional background and qualifications.
- To assist in the personal evaluation of career development, professional involvement, continuing education needs, and publishing record, for example.

COMPILING A CURRICULUM VITAE

The grammar, spelling and general appearance of a CV must be of a high standard. It must be well laid out and pleasing to the eye and generally have a professional appearance. It should therefore be typed by a professional secretary or on a word processor. On *no* account must a handwritten CV be submitted.

There are no absolute guidelines for constructing a CV. A suggested outline from which a structure might be developed follows.

Personal details

Name
Home address
Home telephone
Work address
Work telephone
Citizenship
Date of birth
Present work position

[At this point only the title of the position and place of employment should be included. An outline of the major responsibilities of the position should appear in the body of the CV.]

Educational qualifications

This section must contain, in chronological order, a description of professional and academic qualifications. It may be necessary to include educational qualifications obtained at school, depending on the career point at which the CV is being prepared. They might, for example, be included if an inexperienced person is applying for a first job or for entry to a course where such educational qualifications are important. If an experienced person is applying for a senior position, items included at the beginning of a career may be omitted in favour of more recent and relevant ones. These points underline the fact that individuals make decisions regarding some aspects of content and structure.

Clinical appointments

This section must list, also in chronological order, all clinical appointments since qualifying. The place of work must be included, together with the dates of the appointment and, if appropriate, the name(s) of senior colleague(s). Decisions must be made on whether or not to include further details, for example to indicate that the time was distributed equally between medical and surgical work, or exclusively in rehabilitation or continuing care. The list of clinical appointments continues until the present or most recent position is reached. For example:

July 1981 to April 1983 (position and specialty)
May 1983 to December 1985 (position and specialty)
January 1986 to August 1989 (position and specialty)
September 1989 to present (position and specialty)

Teaching appointments

This part will be of relevance to those who are currently working as teachers/lecturers, or who have worked as such in the past. It is necessary to decide whether or not to include a summary of the major subject areas taught. Thus, if the CV is to accompany an application for a first teaching appointment or for a place on a teaching course, it might be useful to use an alternative subheading, 'Teaching experience'. Entries might, for example, include teaching students in clinical areas or in the classroom, teaching staff from the applicant's own profession and/or from other professions on the in-service education programme, and visiting lectureships at departments of medicine, nursing, physiotherapy, occupational therapy and chiropody.

June 1986 to August 1987: Clinical tutor to 1st year students
April 1987 to March 1988: Director, In-service Education Programme
1989 to present: Regular contributor, approximately monthly, to hospital study-day programme.

Continuing education

This covers participation in courses, study days, conferences, study visits and so on. Unless a note is kept of these items as they occur, there is a strong possibility that they will be overlooked when updating a CV. The applicant has to decide how far back this entry should go. If qualified for a number of years, only entries for the past seven years might, for example, be included and this should be made clear at the start of the section. In some instances a request might be made to include entries for a specified time period, for example that conference presentations and publications should be for only the past five years.

Initially, all relevant information should be recorded in the CV, which can then be edited to suit any occasion. It is important to bear in mind that it might, for example, become necessary to describe a study-day presentation made five years previously. Examples of entries might be:

Conference attendance: 'Research ethics', University of Peel, 1 July 1992

'Advances in surgical care', Finpark General Hospital, 21 April 1991

Short course attendance: 'Rehabilitation of the amputee', Axford Health Centre, 1 June 1986

'Preparing a literature review', Mongton Health Sciences Library, 7–9 September 1986

Professional visits: Adult Medical Unit, Dalton General Hospital, 17 December 1985

Papers presented

A full reference to each paper presented as part of a conference, study day or seminar should be included. The following are examples of entries.

'Multidisciplinary casework'. Health Research in the 1990s, Effingham College, 28 April 1991.

'Anxiety in pre-operative patients'. Issues in General Surgery study day, Georgetown College, 8 November 1989

Publications

A chronological list of all publications in journals, books and published conference proceedings is an integral part of a CV. The more experienced the person, the greater the number of entries expected. Because some organizations distinguish between articles published in refereed journals and those in non-refereed journals, it is necessary to distinguish between the two. This can be done by indicating referenced journals by means of an asterisk.

Publications (= refereed journal)*

Examples of entries (in date order) might be:

*Smith, P. (1985) Wound care in the elderly. *Journal of Health Care* **7** (12) 54–56.

*Smith, P. and Hislopp, J. (1986) Issues relating to mobility. *Journal of Continuing Care* **8** (32) 23–27.

Smith, P. (1988) Cell damage. Letter to *Journal of Tissue Pathology* **5** (11) 12.

Gault, H. and Smith, P. (1992) Issues in general management. *Journal of Health Care Management* **5** (11) 45–51.

Unless asked to do otherwise by the person or organization that requires the CV, all publications must be included.

Related publishing experience, for example book reviews, manuscript review panel membership, or publishing consultancies, should be included in separate sections.

Management experience

In almost every position occupied by a health care professional, including those that are clinical, educational or research based, there is a managerial element. A CV should therefore contain some reference to this area of responsibility. For example, a clinician might write:

1989–1990: [title of position]. In addition to previously specified clinical responsibilities, managerial functions included membership of the Unit Management Team
1991–1992: Clinical co-ordinator for medical area

Research

Details of involvement in any aspect of health care related research must be included here. Useful headings are:

Personal research
Multidisciplinary research projects
Supervision of research done by others
Refereeing research proposals
Research and ethics committee membership
Research grants received

Awards, commendations, prizes and honours

Details of all awards received on a competitive basis must be given, including travel scholarships and research fellowships, honours or prizes.

1986: Collingberg Prize for distinction in the study of pathology of old age, Forthfield University

1987: Phillips Travel Scholarship. Undertook a two-month study tour of rehabilitation units in the USA

Professional organizations/activities

Details of participation in the work of professional organizations constitutes an important and legitimate part of a curriculum vitae. Entries in this section might include:

Member: 1984 [Name of organization]
Chairman: 1986–1987 [Name of organization]
Member: 1989 [Name of specialist society]
Member: 1990 [Name of specialist association]

Community activities

Some employers value the voluntary involvement of staff in health related community work. Indeed, some organizations in North America expect staff to make contributions of this kind. Examples include:

1984–1985: Member, Clarkstone Community Association
1986–1987: Member, Peel Area Health Board
1989–present: Secretary, Mintlock Area Local Health Council

Other items that should be included if appropriate include:

Consultancies
Interdisciplinary/multidisciplinary teaching
External examinerships
External assessor (interviews)
Committee memberships (past and present)
Workshop presentation

GENERAL HINTS ON CV PREPARATION

- A new entrant to a profession should not be concerned that the CV is rather short; it will expand as the career develops.
- When writing a CV it is important to be honest and bold. This is no place for misplaced modesty.
- It must be assumed that a CV will be required sooner rather than later. It is a statement of fact which reflects professional career development. The more professionally active the individual, the more comprehensive it is, and the more recent will be the entries.
- Items for inclusion must be recorded as they occur; they should start at the point of entry into the profession.

- The CV must be professionally written and presented; it must *never* be handwritten. Ideally, a word processor should be used, or a secretary who uses one should be employed.
- If it is not clear as to the section in which a particular item should be placed, the one that seems most appropriate should be chosen. The important thing is to include all relevant information.
- The CV must be short, sharp and to the point.
- Before, during and after preparing a CV it should be discussed with a colleague who has personal experience of CV preparation.
- The content of a CV is likely to be the subject of detailed discussion at interview if it has been submitted in support of an application for a job or travel scholarship, for example. The applicant must therefore be prepared to discuss, defend and justify *every* item in it, and to explain the absence of particular items.
- In order that referees will be able to add their support for something for which a CV is being submitted, they should be sent a copy.
- A curriculum vitae is often the opportunity to make a good first impression. If that opportunity is lost, there is no second chance.

THE RÉSUMÉ

A résumé is a summary of a curriculum vitae and should include all its major headings. Because the CV of a new entrant will be relatively short, there is no need for it to be summarized as a résumé.

The publications section of a résumé might read:

Seven articles/book chapters published since 1985.

Similarly, clinical appointments might be summarized as follows:

1972–1986: Various appointments as [specify grades] and [specify] in [specify specialties].

If asked for a curriculum vitae, it is clear that a full one is required. If a résumé is requested, it may be necessary to clarify whether a full CV or a summary is required. This warning is given in the knowledge that the term 'résumé' is often used by people who actually mean 'curriculum vitae'. If there is still doubt as to which is required, a full personal record should be sent.

Chapter 17
Book Reviews

Book reviewing uses many of the skills required in other forms of writing; for example a clear, concise writing style with which to convey the maximum amount of material using a prescribed and limited number of words. Most health care journals include a section of reviews of recently published texts. They are written by clinicians, educators, researchers or managers recruited by the journal specifically for the task. The people recruited must have the following qualifications: an ability to write concise and informative reviews, a high level of expertise in the subject of the book to be reviewed, and/or membership of the group at which a book is aimed.

WHAT ARE BOOK REVIEWS?

A review is a published critical appraisal of a book. It is written by an independent specialist in the book's subject matter. Books are normally sent by publishers to selected journals, whose review editors then select reviewers. For example, those intended for a multidisciplinary readership will be sent to journals with a similar readership. Those with a specific clinical focus will be sent to journals dealing with that topic. Books that are educational or managerial in emphasis will be sent to educational and managerial journals respectively. Some specialized texts will be sent to specialized *and* wide readership journals.

The purpose of a review is to provide the potential buyer or reader with an independent and specialist opinion of the content and quality of the book. A review will also provide important feedback to the author/editor and the publisher. Thus the reader is relying on the credibility, credentials and expertise of the reviewer who has a responsibility to the journal, to its readership and to the author(s) and publisher of the book.

Journals have varying requirements for the structure and length of a review, and these are given to its writer. The requirements may range from a request to provide a review with a maximum length of 300 words, with no additional instructions; to a request to produce a 200-word opinion that will cover a number of points contained in a specific instruction from the journal.

In general the purpose of a review is:

- To inform the reader of the purpose of the book. It will clearly state what the writer(s) claim the book is intended to do, and whether or not that has been achieved.
- To describe the author(s) or editor(s) or contributors to the book, giving some information about their professional credentials and referring to the country or countries in which they currently work and where the book may have originated.
- To comment on the intended readership as described by the author(s) or editor(s), and to indicate whether or not it is suitable for that readership.
- To give an opinion as to the quality and presentation of the contents, for example its readability, structure, grammar, references, index and appendices, and as to whether the work is of a scholarly and professional nature.
- To avoid giving a 'bad' book a favourable or neutral review, or a 'good' book a poor or neutral one. These are the cardinal sins of book reviewing.
- To comment on whether or not the book represents value for money.
- To compare the book with its competitors, if there are any on the market.
- To indicate whether or not the book is up to date.
- To make a firm statement that will help the reader decide whether to examine the book, buy one for personal use or have a library copy bought.

Although this is a task that carries a considerable amount of responsibility, it is a rewarding, informative and challenging means of keeping up to date with a specialist area. At the same time it enables the reviewer to play a part in developing a health care profession with its own distinct literature. Book reviewing is not for the fainthearted, indecisive or over-sensitive since it often demands the use of tough decisions and language.

WHO COMMISSIONS BOOK REVIEWS?

To ensure that a review is impartial, unbiased and objective, the reviewer is recruited by the journal in which the review is to be published rather than by the book publisher. The book review editor of the journal will have a list of names of well qualified individuals to whom books can be sent. Thus if a book relating to post-surgical rehabilitation of the elderly is received, it will be sent to a specialist in that subject. If the recipient feels, for any reason, unwilling or unable to review a book, it should be returned immediately to the journal with a note of explanation. For example, the subject of the text might be outside the reviewer's competence, or they might have personal links with the author and feel that this could prevent them from expressing a wholly unbiased opinion. Thus there is always the right to accept or refuse an invitation to review.

WHO WRITES BOOK REVIEWS?

The major requirement for reviewing is that the reviewer be an experienced professional in either a number of areas or in a single specialism. The experience of the potential reviewer will determine the types of book he or she is qualified to deal with. For example, if a person has a wide experience of many areas of health care, reviewing books on a range of topics would be appropriate. Conversely, if experience is highly specialized, reviewing might be limited to that topic. What is being indicated here is that the reviewing system requires a wide range of professional experience and backgrounds in health care professionals who are to become reviewers.

Another prerequisite is that the potential reviewer should have the skill necessary to meet the requirements of the review and of the journal that requests it. People who review books may have moved into this area of publication having previously gained experience in, for example, writing articles or books or both. However, there is no reason why reviewing should not be a first publishing experience.

BECOMING A BOOK REVIEWER

There are a number of ways of becoming a reviewer. First, individuals might be contacted by a journal editor who knows them to have the necessary skill and professional expertise. This type of contact depends on the editor knowing or having been informed of the suitability of the people concerned. This might be the case when the editor contacts a potential reviewer who is well established and well known for professional expertise.

Another method of recruitment, particularly by new journals, is for the review editor to place an advertisement in the journal inviting potential reviewers to apply. This means of recruiting reviewers is less commonly employed than others.

The third method depends on an initiative being taken by people who wish to become reviewers. Some may be reluctant to take such an initiative; nevertheless, this is acceptable and common. Here the potential reviewer writes to the journal editor enclosing a letter and curriculum vitae designed to invite the editor to consider using him or her. The letter should be positive and persuasive, and contain a full description of the writer's experience and expertise. The journal's review editor will want to be convinced that the applicant has something special to offer. It might be worth while enclosing a well written and informative sample review of a text which is within the aspiring reviewer's expertise. The request to become a reviewer might be accepted or rejected. If rejected this may be because the journal already has sufficient reviewers in the subject area. There is no need to feel discouraged by rejection; a similar application should simply be made to another appropriate journal.

WRITING THE REVIEW

The reviewer should start with two pages of paper and write the topics to be covered in the review, leaving enough space between each for the actual review material. The preface, foreword and further details of the book, which usually appear on the back cover, should be read. These items should summarize the aim, content and intended readership. If, after reading the book, a reviewer disagrees with any of the claims made about the book by the author/editor who writes the preface and the entry on the back cover, or with the foreword which is written by someone recruited by the writer of the book, this should be clearly stated and explained.

The book must then be read in its entirety and notes must be entered in the appropriate sections of the review outline. Writing a second and third draft enables improvements in style and brevity to be made. Particular attention must be paid to length, which is *never* more than the maximum requested. The review must then be typed according to the guide provided by the journal, usually in double spacing, and sent off.

The fictional Example 40 which follows is approximately 350 words long and would be quite adequate in response to a request for a 400-word maximum length. The headings in italics are for guidance only and do not appear in the review. The material under each heading is an example of a review.

Example 40 _____

Book Review

Book title
    Community Care of the Elderly: A Political Perspective
Aims and intended readership
        Presents a multidisciplinary view of the social and political
        structures needed to provide community care for the elderly in
        Great Britain. It is written for staff of all disciplines involved in
        planning for and providing this type of care.
Brief details of author(s), editor(s)
        The 14 contributors, all well qualified and well known in their
        fields, are drawn from the major disciplines involved in
        managing and providing community care in Great Britain.

Outline of content/chapters

    The book has three parts. The first, with three chapters, deals with the general history and politics of the development of community care. Part 2 has nine chapters, each presenting the topic from the viewpoint of each of the disciplines involved in care management and delivery. Part 3 contains chapters written by a member of parliament, a clinician, a health care manager and a director of social work, each of whom speculates about the future.

Index, appendices, figures and tables

    The index, 24 tables and figures and the appendices are well presented and informative.

Quality and level of content (introductory or advanced)

    The level of the book makes it suitable for senior students in all disciplines and for qualified staff who need to update themselves.

Presentation and readability

    The book is well presented and readable. As expected with a multiauthor book, there is variability in style and presentation. However, the editor has ensured that this does not detract from the high quality of this work in terms of consistency, style, fluency and presentation.

Academic quality

    Academically the book is of high quality and is appropriate to the subject and the book's readership.

Up to date or not

    The content is current and makes reference to all recent legislation and major developments.

Comparison with competitor books

    It generally compares favourably with the small number of other books on the same subject.

Value for money

    Community Care of the Elderly: A Political Perspective represents excellent value for money.

Reviewer's recommended readership

    It is well suited to its intended readership.

Suggest purchase of personal and/or library copies

    All health care libraries should buy a copy and all health care students should have access to a copy for general/reference use; students on specialist community courses will benefit from owning a copy.

Concluding/summary statement

    This is an excellent book which I have no hesitation in recommending to students and qualified staff in all health care professions.

AFTER PUBLICATION

Although reviews can have a considerable impact on the professional and literary reputation of authors and editors, and there may be major financial consequences for those who wrote and published the book, all expect reviewers to produce a frank and balanced opinion. In particular, review readers depend on the objectivity and honesty of the reviewer.

In most instances the work of the reviewer, in relation to a particular book, ends with publication of the review. However, there may be instances in which discussion, compliment or criticism of the review may occur, or where agreement or disagreement may be voiced. For example, the journal publishing the review may subsequently carry Letters to the Editor commenting on the content of a recently published review. These letters come from a number of sources, including the author or editor of the book, or journal readers who disagree with the review. In any event book reviewers who have done their job well have little to fear from those who disagree.

PAYMENT OF BOOK REVIEWERS

The payment offered to reviewers differs between journals. If payment is made, it is of a token nature and does not cover the full cost of typing, time and materials. Thus book reviewing, as with many aspects of professional writing, cannot be seen as an income-generating activity but rather as an opportunity to participate in the development of a literature base for the health care professions.

If payment is made it is usually one of two types: first, payment in the form of being able to retain the reviewed book, which will be of variable value; secondly, payment in the form of a *very* small fee and retention of the book.

Chapter 18
Writing and Presenting a Speech

The term 'speech' refers to the presentation of papers at conferences, study days and seminars, to giving a talk or presentation, and to public speaking. The formality or informality of the talk depends on its purpose, the audience, and where it is delivered. The general principles that apply to this form of writing apply equally to the large formal presentation and to the small informal one (a lunchtime case presentation, for example). The informal talk is similar in some ways to classroom teaching or to the presentation of discussion papers within a classroom. Writing for those two forms of public speaking which are more aligned to teaching will not be discussed in this chapter, although some of the principles are obviously the same. Because writing a speech is closely linked to its presentation, both aspects are discussed in this chapter.

Professional success is undoubtedly enhanced by an ability to communicate (formally or informally) with large or small groups such as those attending study days and conferences. Examples are: the researcher who presents findings to a conference; the clinician describing a newly developed technique at a local study day; the clinical manager explaining managerial changes to a large audience at a hospital-based seminar; and the teacher presenting a paper at a local education seminar. Contributions of this kind from all professions are now the rule rather than the exception. Professionals present papers for a variety of reasons: first, to respond to the needs of others for information; secondly, to enhance personal career development in terms of providing experience in what will become a normal part of everyday duties; and thirdly, in order to contribute to the exchange of information, a vital component of the work of health care professionals.

Prior to writing a talk the beginner will understandably ask: 'Can I do it, and do I have anything to say?'

CAN I TALK IN PUBLIC?

For all professionals the answer is 'yes', if they want to. All have something important to say, although some underestimate the ability to do so. This position is analogous to that encountered in Sweden in relation to the use which young Swedes made (or did not make) of

English lessons received in school. Many Swedes were reluctant to use their English in public for fear of making mistakes. However, once they took the plunge and got started, there was no looking back. The fear of failure, which can be very strong, is overcome by good preparation, starting with relatively small and informal engagements, and by knowing that speaking in public comes naturally to some and can be learned by others. It is, of course, a responsibility of all members of all professions. Failure to develop this form of writing and presentation skill can be a very serious professional impediment.

WHERE DO I BEGIN?

Many opportunities exist, both during and immediately after basic professional education, to develop speaking skills. They include writing and presenting class discussion papers, teaching practice with fellow students, contributing to in-service training, presentations at hospital study days, and contributing to a group paper at a local conference. Opportunities can also be created by, for example, getting together with others who wish to develop public speaking skills and constructing an in-service programme specifically designed to give the chance to present a paper to the rest of the group for constructive criticism. Such a programme, involving one participant with public speaking experience, can help beginners to get started. Senior colleagues with experience in public speaking, from any discipline, are well qualified to help inexperienced colleagues develop these skills. Some health care conferences actively encourage some first-time speakers. With assistance and support from conference organizers and colleagues generally, this can help to enlarge considerably the pool of public speaking skills available within the health care system.

Speakers are generally invited for one of two reasons. The first is that the individual is of a very high standing within the profession and will undoubtedly say something of interest whatever the topic covered. Such speakers are often given a relatively open invitation to speak on a topic of their choosing. For example, the invitation might be to present the opening address at the start of a conference. More commonly, certainly in numerical terms, people are invited to speak on a particular subject within their area of expertise. Although there is often some room for negotiation in terms of the precise nature of the subject, or of the title to be used, these invitations usually relate to a specific topic. Examples might be: a clinician invited to talk about pre-operative anxiety; a researcher about the subject of a research study such as 'The prevention of pressure sores in the terminally ill'; a manager about means of monitoring staff sickness and absence levels; and an educator about developments in computer-assisted learning.

An alternative to a personal invitation is to respond to a 'Call for Abstracts' which is a general invitation from conference organizers to possible speakers to send an abstract of a paper they would like to present. The structure of the 'Call for Abstracts' (see Example 41) indicates the criteria on which abstracts will be judged. Usually, but not always, requests for abstracts are found in professional journals.

Example 41

Call for Abstracts

'Post-traumatic rehabilitation of children:
recent research and research applications'
Rehabilitation Unit, Fairfax Memorial Hospital
(See accompanying advertisement for full conference details)

1. Clinicians and researchers are invited to submit abstracts on all relevant aspects of the subject of the conference. In addition to research papers, contributions are also invited from clinicians who wish to demonstrate the application of clinical research.
2. Speakers will each be allocated 45 minutes for the presentation, including 15 minutes for discussion.
3. Abstracts will be considered by the conference abstracts group, who will judge whether or not the abstract meets the requirements of the conference. The closing date for submission of abstracts is 14 January 1994.
4. Abstracts should be submitted to The Conference Secretary, Room 112, Fairfax Memorial Hospital.

Abstract format
Abstracts should be typed in double spacing on no more than two sheets of typescript.

Sheet 1:	(i)	Paper title (maximum of eight words)
	(ii)	Name and qualifications of the author
	(iii)	Business address
	(iv)	Home and business telephone numbers
	(v)	Present work position
	(vi)	Audio-visual requirements
Sheet 2:	(vii)	Abstract, 200 words maximum

The abstract will state the aims and outcome of a research study and/or clearly demonstrate the application of research to clinical work.

INVITATION TO PRESENT A PAPER

Someone with acknowledged expertise in the subject of the conference might be invited to give a talk without first having to submit an abstract. If such an invitation is received, the following questions must be considered before deciding whether to accept or refuse it.

Can I do it? Usually, the person extending the invitation will have done their homework first. However, it is not unheard of for individuals to get an invitation to speak on a subject which is not their area of expertise, or with which they are now out of touch. If justice cannot be done to the invitation, it should be refused immediately and a reason given. The recipient should not be tempted to accept because a refusal might inconvenience the conference organizers, or because it would provide filler for a curriculum vitae. Experienced *and* novice speakers must be discerning about when to accept and when to refuse invitations.

General content. An invitation will include general guidelines such as the subject of the presentation, 'The pathology of pressure sores' for example. More detailed guidelines might be to speak about the prevention of pressure sores in the 1990s in relation to the unconscious patient. At this point it might be possible to negotiate a slight change in the focus of the paper, with the organizers agreeing to the appropriate exclusion or inclusion of material. There is no need to feel reluctant to negotiate the nature and content of an invited paper, as long as this is done early on.

Who will I be speaking to? An idea of the audience size, and of the background of those attending, will establish if a talk can be prepared to meet the needs of this particular audience.

Will conference papers be published/circulated? Papers read at some conferences are formally published by the organizers. On other occasions they might be circulated to participants after the conference. Speakers need to know about such arrangements well in advance to enable them to prepare a paper for others to read. There is a considerable difference between a paper which is prepared for reading and subsequent publication or distribution to others, and one intended for use only for presentation at a conference. Although it is usual for organizers to give fair notice of these arrangements, speakers might be asked to transfer rough notes into a publishable paper at short notice. Even if the paper is not to be published by the conference organizers, the writer should seriously consider revamping it for submission to a professional journal (see Chapter 15). If the decision to publish is taken prior to the conference date, a colleague should be asked to take notes on the discussion of the paper; details can then be included in the published version.

The speaking fee and travel and subsistence costs should be discussed with the organizer as early as possible. A fee may be offered or the speaker may be asked whether one is charged and, if so, how much. One possible reply is that there is no fee but reimbursement of travelling and living expenses is expected. The payment of fees and costs is an individual matter which the speaker and conference organizers must negotiate.

WRITING THE PAPER

Those preparing a paper for the first time should begin the work well in advance. They should start by researching and reading around the subject to update and extend knowledge of it. Many papers include some material written by other people, one reviewing research of the subject area, for example, and must include full references and acknowledgements. If references are used, they must be typed up and duplicated and a copy must be given to each conference participant as they will *not* be able to take a full note of references during the talk.

The writer should start developing the paper by making rough notes of key words and phrases, then arranging them into sequence. The rough notes form the basis of the paper which will go through a number of drafts before the final one is ready. As the paper develops, the speaker must estimate how long it should be to fill the allocated time. If committing every word to paper, a method used by some speakers, it is necessary to determine how many words, or how many pages of double-spaced typescript, equate to a 20-minute talk, for example. This can be done by measuring how long it takes to read aloud one page typed in double spacing, calculating the number of pages that can be read in the allocated time, then writing a talk of the desired length. It should be borne in mind that reading a page of script silently takes far less time than it takes to read the same page aloud to an audience. A paper should *never* be too long; if in doubt, it should be shortened. An audience and chairperson will be forgiving if a speaker finishes slightly early; both may become restless if the agreed time is exceeded. Worse still, it can be very difficult if, half-way through the paper, the chairperson suddenly announces that 'Your 20 minutes are up and you now have to stop', or 'You now have one minute to go', and there are still five unread pages. Speakers who go over their allotted time take a considerable risk and may be regarded as unprofessional.

KEY DECISIONS

As the paper develops, a number of decisions must be made that have implications for its format, content and structure.

Questions are usually taken at the end of the talk, although some speakers prefer them to be raised during an informal talk. The decision is a matter for discussion between the speaker and the chairman of the session. It must be decided as to when to allow questions and how much time should be devoted to these and to discussion if both are to be dealt with at the end. For example, a 30-minute paper may allow for 20 minutes' presentation and 10 minutes' discussion. If the allotted time includes question/discussion time, both audience and speaker should be aware of what the arrangements are and that they must be adhered to.

Audio-visual aids (slides or a video, for example) might be used either as a means of adding variety to a talk, or as a key part of it. If they are to be used, the speaker should consider getting advice from an audio-visual aids department. The aids should be tested in advance of the conference day, and a check must be made that equipment is available for their use.

The *structure of notes* depends on experience and on the planned formality or informality of the speech. Detailed notes may be typed, in double spacing, on 15 cm × 10 cm (6 in × 4 in) cards or on A4-size paper. Whichever format is used, a page or card number should be written clearly on the front of each item in case they become mixed up before or (worse still) during the talk. For some speakers, particularly beginners, verbatim notes might be preferred. Alternatively notes can be prepared in the form of topics, headings, prompts and personal cues; this approach is the one more favoured by the experienced speaker, particularly on less formal occasions.

Some speakers deliver a talk without notes. They are either brave or naive, and usually either very good or very, very bad. It is vital to have some form of notes at hand although these may be used less frequently with experience and confidence.

In addition to the substance of the talk, notes contain prompts which form a guide during delivery. They might be written in red ink, at the points in the talk where reminders are needed. For example:

- Make sure watch and drinking water on table.
- Show first slide here.
- Check that audience can read it.
- Check that the people at the back can still hear (repeated four times in talk).
- Check that half-way stage (10.30) is reached.
- Refer to handout No. 1.
- Present second slide.

DEVELOPING THE WRITTEN PAPER

Now that the general structure and format of the talk are ready, the full paper must be written. As the content of papers varies, only the general principles of structure are covered here.

Preliminary material

Each speaker is introduced by a chairperson who chairs either the entire conference, part of it, or an individual paper. The job of the chairperson is to present the speaker, having earlier obtained details about their professional experiences and background by asking for a résumé.

In terms of *structure* the first part of the paper might include the following.

- *Thanking the chairperson* for the introduction: a useful opener which helps to get started, then thanking the person who extended the invitation to speak at the conference.
- *Personal details*, in addition to those given by the chair. For example, if previous experience includes working with deaf children and this is relevant to the paper, the audience should be informed.
- *Brief social chat* will help form a rapport with the audience and might include such informal comments as the pleasure obtained from visiting the particular institution or city.
- *Administrative details* of the talk, unless announced by the chair, can be given here. For example, the audience might be reminded that there will be a 20-minute talk followed by 10 minutes for discussion. If handouts have been distributed to the audience, it is important to ensure that everyone has a copy before starting.
- *The title and summary of the paper* are then given, even if the title has already been stated by the chair. For example, after the title the speaker might say: 'In the first part of this paper I will present an outline of the clinical responsibilities of the multidisciplinary team in the unit in which I work. Next, I will discuss my role in detail, and its relationship to the work of other team members. Finally, I will discuss plans for developing the unit during the next five years.' This summary prepares the audience for what is to follow, and it helps them to digest and remember the substance of the paper.

The talk

The body of the talk follows the summary, and constitutes the bulk of the paper. In writing the speech, full use should be made of major headings, subheadings and sub-subheadings. Although the audience does not see them, they can be used to indicate when new topics are being moved on to, or where a subtopic is part of a major topic. Below headings it may be useful to include statements such as 'Now I will move on to consider the advantages of that approach'. These techniques will help in the preparation of a logical and coherent paper that can be read in a relaxed and unhurried way.

The concluding section draws the paper to a close and reminds the audience of the major topics covered in the paper. An example might be: 'In conclusion, I have covered the following topics . . .'. This prompts the audience to expect the talk to finish soon, and to anticipate, and prepare to respond to, a final concluding statement such as 'Thank you very much for giving me this opportunity to come here today to discuss . . .'.

ARRIVAL AT THE CONFERENCE VENUE

If possible, preparations for the presentation should continue after arrival at the conference venue.

- The speaker should *visit the hall or room* where the paper will be read and get a feel for it.
- *Audio-visual aids*, particularly the microphone, must be tested. If a microphone is not being used, the speaker should ask someone to stand at the back of the room and indicate whether they can hear a medium-level voice. The speaker must not shout as this cannot be sustained for a 20- or 30-minute talk. If aids such as a slide or overhead projector are being used, the speaker must find out who will operate them, who will adjust the lights and open and close curtains, and who (if anyone) will be available to assist if things go wrong. It is best to assume that the conference organizers might possibly overlook something.
- It is important to *check the platform props* and, if necessary, to alter the position of the table, chair, microphone and lectern, for example. The height of the lectern must be checked. If there is no lectern, the speaker will have to decide where to place notes when speaking. He or she should also ensure that a jug of water and a glass are available.

Reading the paper

Prior to presentation all speakers feel nervous; this is natural. However, rehearsed and well prepared notes will give confidence, and the inserted cues and prompts will provide additional familiar landmarks and natural breaks. The speaker should *never* begin a presentation with a polite apology for inexperience even if this is the first time he or she has spoken in public. It is absolutely unnecessary and detracts from the quality of the paper. Nervousness is something about which speakers are much more aware than are audiences.

Notes should indicate what to say and include prompts such as 'check they can hear at the back' or an emphasized word or phrase written in BLOCK CAPITALS, or underlined. The speaker should also use appropriate variation in tone and speed to give emphasis, animated body language, and brief eye contact with a number of participants. Some techniques (such as inserting comments and cues in notes) may help. For example, key words can be highlighted in notes, points to be emphasized can be underlined and capital letters and spaces can be used to indicate where to aim for dramatic effect. Personal instructions, such as 'pause', should be noted; these prompts will guide presentation of the material. An example is:

'Pressure sores <u>can be prevented</u> in most cases. Consider the range of preventive measures described in the research literature. Consider the application (or otherwise) of these measures. [PAUSE] I propose that we <u>can</u> do more with increased equipment budgets.'

Experience enables a speaker to accommodate spontaneous responses such as applause from the audience, and to know when to inject pauses to let a point 'sink in'. Body language should be used to enable communication with the audience. Experienced speakers make good use of non-verbal cues. One example is gaining attention by standing up straight and getting eye contact when talking. Conversely, when talking with a small informal group, the speaker's contribution to discussion might be improved by sitting down and adopting a relatively passive posture.

A firm understanding of the subject of the speech will give confidence and enable less use to be made of notes than might have been anticipated, or even deviation from them when appropriate. Initially, speakers usually prefer detailed notes and are most comfortable when reading directly from them when speaking. Experience will enable concentration on style of presentation in addition to content.

Time spent in planning the content and structure of notes will assist presentation. Earlier practice at reading and timing the material aloud, to a friend or into a tape recorder, helps a lot. 'Practice runs' help produce a conversational style of presentation.

The arrangement made with the chairperson will decide how 'question time' should be handled. The chairperson may invite questions and generally 'control' question time, or the questions might be directed straight to the speaker. Although the vast majority of questions are clear and appropriate, a few are vague and almost meaningless.

For beginners, it is probably best that questions be directed to the chair who will be able, if required, to support the speaker. However, speakers should bear in mind that they are there because they almost certainly know more about the subject of the talk than most of the audience. When receiving and answering questions it is important:

- to accept the questioner's point of view, even if intending to express a different one;
- to ask for clarification if a question is unclear;
- if the answer to a specific question is not known, to say so;
- to redirect questions to the audience if it is felt that someone there may have an answer;
- to accept personal limitations, remembering that nobody has all the answers;
- not to get involved in a long discussion with one person in the audience.

The give and take of question and discussion time is an important part of a talk, as much a learning experience for the speaker as for the audience.

Although public speaking is never entirely free of some anxiety, it does become easier and more enjoyable with experience. One thing which produces most anxiety is the struggle to reach 'perfection', an impossible goal. There is no absolutely 'correct' way of writing and presenting a paper, although there are some useful general principles such as those discussed in this chapter. Because speakers are all individuals with particular strengths and weaknesses, each should use an individual style of delivery, rather than that of a 'model' public speaker.

As with other aspects of writing, the preparation of presentations is the responsibility of every professional. It is best to start with relatively 'easy' topics and short presentations. It may be helpful to manufacture public speaking opportunities, as part of an in-service training programme for example.

The speaker must decide on the overall approach or approaches that will need to be used in the talk, for example information presentation, exploration of issues, discussion of provocative or contentious themes, speculation about future developments, or a combination of these. It may be that the remit from the organizers will indicate the general approach to be used.

When writing and presenting a paper, the speaker should do so in the certain knowledge that the organizers and audience value what they have to say. It is important to write and speak with confidence and enthusiasm.

Practice gained by reading the paper aloud using a mirror is useful. The speaker should move around the 'stage' a little whilst continuing to face the audience. This is the time to practise projecting the voice and developing a delivery style. The use of an empty hall or large room, with a colleague at the back, is another way of testing delivery. The colleague should be asked to comment on the talk. These exercises are valuable ways of testing the amount of time required to deliver a talk. Prior to giving the talk the speaker needs to prepare the stage and the props to enable comfortable communication with the audience. It is important for the speaker to convey that they are in charge of the stage. The talk must be kept simple in terms of sentence construction and general clarity of ideas. Unlike a reader's words, those of a listener cannot be read and reread until the meaning is clear. A real effort is required in order to avoid vague, even rambling, sentences and paragraphs. It is vital to ensure that every word used is likely to be understood by the audience. The speaker must be short, sharp, crisp and to the point, and there must be an understandable and logical flow of ideas. There needs to be less concern about perfect grammar than about conveying ideas and ensuring that they are understood.

Finally, when next attending a study day or conference, or listening to some other form of public talk, it will be helpful to pay particular attention to the *style* of presentation (rather than the content) of some of the talks. Notes should be taken about those aspects of presentation that added to the quality of the speech generally and clarified specific aspects of content. In this way it is possible to add to one's repertoire of successful public speaking techniques.

Chapter 19
Writing a Research Proposal

A research proposal is a structured and detailed description of a proposed piece of research. Although the amount of detail in the proposal submitted by the researcher to others may vary, the researcher personally makes use of all the material described in this chapter. If necessary, the material can be edited, condensed and rearranged to meet the requirements of others such as funding bodies or ethics committees.

In addition to providing a research outline for use by the researcher, and to satisfy the needs of a range of other individuals and groups, the very act of writing the proposal prompts its writer to commit to paper a clear, specific and well argued plan of a complex activity, that is, the proposed research. If there are weaknesses in the planned research, earlier drafts of the proposal will usually reveal these and prompt suitable action.

WHO WRITES THE PROPOSAL?

The proposal, which usually progresses through a number of drafts, is invariably written by the person or persons who will carry out the research. The individual researcher, or research team, takes full responsibility for the proposal content and for ensuring that the subsequent research adheres to the final proposal.

In the case of commissioned research, when another person requests that research be conducted on a specific subject, the researcher may be given the research question or problem only and will construct the remainder of the proposal. Alternatively, the commissioning body may provide the researcher with a more or less complete proposal.

Constructing and subsequently modifying a proposal takes considerable time and includes activities that are part of the actual study, for example undertaking a preliminary search and review of the literature. Working on a full-time basis it would not be unusual for two to four months to be spent on creating a proposal for a moderately large research project.

The role of the research supervisor in the construction of a proposal is crucial, particularly if the proposed research is to be undertaken by a novice. The supervisor guides and advises the person writing the proposal; indeed it is not submitted to the body for which it was prepared until the supervisor is satisfied with it. Many funding, academic and other bodies will only accept a proposal from a beginner if this has been approved and signed by a supervisor who is an experienced researcher.

WHEN IS A PROPOSAL NEEDED?

In addition to meeting the needs of the researcher for a blueprint to work from and acting as a prompt to clear and structured thinking, the proposal is used, possibly in a shortened or modified form, for other purposes.

Funding bodies

Research funding bodies invariably request that a full proposal accompany a request for financial assistance. Some provide applicants with a form requesting specific details of the proposal; others leave the applicant to decide what to include.

Employers

Some employers give staff a reduced workload in order to undertake research. An application for such a reduction by clinicians, managers or teaching staff will invariably have to be accompanied by a proposal that includes an indication of the amount of time off being requested.

Higher-degree registration

Part of the requirement for registering for a higher degree such as Master of Philosophy and Doctor of Philosophy is the submission of a proposal which meets the standards and format of the degree-awarding body. The proposal may have to accompany the registration application, or be submitted and considered at a later date. In either event, the proposal is a key factor in obtaining registration.

Research and Ethics Committee

Many research projects undertaken by health care staff, particularly if they involve collecting data from or about human subjects, are required to be submitted to, and considered and approved by, the Research and Ethics Committee which usually operates within the area for which the local health care system has responsibility. The committee will have to satisfy itself on a number of issues including that:

- the researcher(s) has the ability, qualifications and experience to undertake the research;
- the research design is appropriate to the aims of the research;
- all ethical issues pertaining to the research have been fully and satisfactorily addressed;
- subjects will give free and informed consent;
- if confidentiality and anonymity are promised, the committee will also need to know how this will be achieved.

The section of the proposal dealing with ethical issues, although of particular interest to the Research and Ethics Committee, will also be relevant to all who make use of the proposal.

Gaining access to the research site

Permission needs to be obtained to collect research data, particularly if human subjects are involved or if data are being collected from confidential documents. Those with clinical and/or managerial responsibility for the areas (sites) in which it is proposed to collect data may request a copy of the full proposal in order that a decision can be made to give or withhold permission.

Coursework

A specialized form of research proposal is that prepared as a coursework requirement without subsequent implementation of the proposal in terms of actually doing the research. In this instance, the proposal may be much longer and more detailed than one written for any of the other purposes indicated earlier in this chapter. The length and format of a proposal written for coursework purposes will usually be prescribed by the institution for which the work is being prepared.

PROPOSAL STRUCTURE

The structure of the proposal used by the researcher to guide the project through all its phases must be both detailed and comprehensive. The structure in Example 42 reflects that requirement and, if used for other purposes such as application for funding or reduction in workload, can be modified to comply with the specific requirements of the body to which it is being submitted. It is *not* the case that full details of all aspects of the proposal are used on all occasions.

Example 42   _____

Structure of research proposal

> Title of research
> Name, position and qualifications of researcher(s)
> Collaborating institution, if any
> Overview
> Research question, problem or hypothesis
> Literature review (summary)
> Rationale for research
> Access to research site
> Research design
> Pilot study (if any)
> Sampling of subjects
> Data collection methods
> Data storage
> Data analysis
> Ethical issues
> Application of research findings
> Available resources
> Budget requirements
> Expected timetable
> Supervision
> Names of referees
> Signatures
> Enclosures

Title

As with the title of any piece of written work, the proposal title should be short, clear and descriptive. Although some aspects of a project may alter during its execution, the title should remain essentially unchanged unless the project is abandoned in favour of another one.

Name, position and qualifications

Although included in the curriculum vitae(s) which may accompany the proposal, this information must be given in the early part of the proposal in order that its readers will be able to judge all other information knowing something of the proposal author(s).

Collaborating institutions

The name(s) of any institutions or organizations (including place of work) committed to collaborating in the study must be provided. Collaboration might take the form of providing resources or supervision, access to data, or time to do the research. This information is particularly useful when seeking support from a funding body.

Overview

A brief overview of the proposed study, of about 200 words, will help the proposal's readers to understand subsequent material.

Research question, problem or hypothesis

A concise statement of the research question, or the problem which the research is designed to answer, or the hypothesis (if any) to be tested must be included here.

Literature review

A brief review of a small amount of selected seminal literature will place the proposal study in the context of previous research and non-research publications. This section need not be more than about 100 words long.

Rationale for research

This section should consist of a short, convincing description of the need for the research to be done. A description of what stimulated interest in this particular topic should be included.

Access to research site

The places where it is intended that data will be collected must be identified, and from whom, if people will be involved. The positions of people and the organizations from whom permission will be sought must be indicated.

Research design

It is necessary to provide an overview of the general design to be used, for example experimental or descriptive, historical, action or evaluation, and some detail of the nature and sequence of major points should be given.

Pilot study

If a pilot study is planned, this must be described and details included of the data that will be collected, where and from whom, and how it will be analysed.

Sampling of subjects

Unless an entire population is used (all hospitals in a given geographical area for example), it may be that the population will be representatively sampled using one of a number of named techniques. Alternatively, some other form of subject selection must be identified and discussed.

Data collection methods

Here, the names of the data collection methods must be given. Examples include non-participant observation, structured interview, questionnaire or the critical incident technique. The qualitative and/or quantitative nature of data should be made clear.

Data storage

The methods to be used to store data must be listed; examples include storage in the original format, Copeland–Chatterson cards or a computer.

Data analysis

This section must describe the data analysing techniques to be used and whether these will be qualitative or quantitative or both. If the latter, it is necessary to mention whether descriptive and/or inferential statistics will be used. If the latter, the inferential statistical tests to be used must be stated.

Ethical issues

If the proposed research has no ethical aspects that require discussion, this must be clearly stated. If there are ethical issues inherent in the proposed research, these must be discussed sufficiently fully to convince readers of the proposal that the researcher is fully aware of them, and that the research design deals appropriately with them and ensures that subjects of the research will be fully protected. The issues of confidentiality and anonymity will feature here.

Application of research findings

Here, the anticipated clinical, managerial or educational significance of the proposed research must be specified. It may be necessary to emphasize a selected applied aspect of the work in order to meet the requirements of a recipient, a body that specializes in funding educational research for example or another whose primary focus is clinical research.

Available resources

Here, the resources (if any) that are already available to support the proposed research must be indicated. Examples include library facilities, inter-library loans, photocopying, statistical advice, printing, computer time, secretarial help and so on.

Budget requirements

This part may only be required if applying for funds to support a project. Funding bodies will want to know which resources already exist to support the work (see preceding section) and which, with costs, are being requested. Examples include:

- Salary/salaries, e.g. researcher, data collector(s). Salaries and related costs are best calculated in consultation with a senior member of the finance department.
- Office space, heating, lighting, cleaning, etc.
- Equipment, e.g. tape recorder, word processor, laboratory hardware. Equipment repairs and insurance costs may have to be met.
- Stationery, e.g. envelopes and paper.
- Inter-library loans.
- Books and journals.
- Printing.
- Postage.
- Specialist advice, e.g. statistics and computing.
- Travel and subsistence costs, e.g. to collect data and/or to meet with other researchers or experts in the subject.
- Conference attendance: fees, travel and subsistence costs.
- Computer time.
- On-line literature search.

Expected timetable

This will show how the total anticipated duration of the proposed research will be distributed between its various parts. The first step is to decide on the length of the project, a decision influenced by the time available to the researcher and the time needed to do the research. Once this is known, time is allocated to the proposal parts which might include those in Example 43.

Supervision

The name and sometimes the signature of the supervisor are requested on many proposal forms. The curriculum vitae of the supervisor may also be requested.

Example 43 _____

Structure of research project timetable

Literature search
Writing up literature review
Refining research design
Gaining access to research site
Selecting and refining data collection instruments
   Pilot study
     Testing data collection instruments
     Storing pilot data
     Analysing pilot data
Modifying research design (if necessary)
Collecting data for main study
Storing data from main study
Analysing data from main study
Writing research report

Names of referees

In some instances the name of one or more referees is required, for example when funding is being requested or if the proposal is for higher-degree registration. The recipient of the proposal will expect the referee to be a competent researcher and/or be someone who knows the professional competence of the proposal writer, and to be familiar with the proposal and its subject matter. The writer of the proposal will hope that the referee is supportive, and no doubt select accordingly.

Enclosures

Some bodies expressly request that no enclosures accompany a proposal, others require them, and still others leave it up to the discretion of the writer. Those included, when appropriate, are the curriculum vitae of the writer(s) and supervisor(s), a list of any references to the literature included in the proposal, and letters of support from a collaborating institution.

GENERAL HINTS

- The proposal and the enclosures must be prepared in high quality typescript, preferably using a word processor.
- The writer must personally ensure that there are no errors of any kind, then ask someone else to proofread the material.
- It is important to make sure that the research design section is particularly clear, specific and appropriate to the aims of the research.

- Except when discussing matters that have already occurred (offers of resources and published literature referred to in the proposal, for example), the future tense must be used consistently throughout.
- Although a full and detailed proposal is a necessary and useful working blueprint for the researcher, it will almost certainly have to be shortened and modified prior to submission to one or other of the many bodies who are recipients of proposals. If the length is constrained through the provision of a form of limited length only essential additional material must be included *if permitted*.

Chapter 20
Travel Scholarship Applications

A number of travel scholarships, often referred to as travel fellowships, are available to the health care professions. They provide excellent opportunities for developing a career in a unique way, and for generating publishable material. The scholarships discussed here are those that enable people to travel (usually abroad) to study or participate in a well defined area of clinical practice, research, management or education. They might, for example, enable a visit to centres of excellence overseas to study the organization of a specialty on a national basis, or to look at new techniques for the care of diabetic children, for patient assessment or for the preparation of multidisciplinary case notes, or to study the use of information technology in health care education. Although all professionals benefit from this type of experience, some may not be aware of the range of opportunities that exist or may have difficulty with the structure or content of an application. Given the large number of health care professionals and the relatively small number of available scholarships, competition is great. Very often, a well written application is the key that opens the door to an interview and possibly a scholarship award.

TRAVEL SCHOLARSHIP TYPES

The types of travel scholarship range from local or regional ones in which staff in a specific geographical area are eligible, to national or international ones with a much wider eligibility. Local scholarships might finance one or two people per year, the large ones many more. Some are funded by charitable donations, others by commercial organizations, and yet others by professional bodies and trade unions.

Via the scholarships, funding organizations contribute generally to the development of the health professions or of a specific discipline or staff grade within it, or might focus on the care of a particular patient diagnostic group. This is achieved by financing people with the intention of developing them individually and through them their profession and health care generally. The long-standing availability of scholarships results from the acknowledgement of the ease with which health care principles are readily transferable between countries and cultures.

Because the cost of such an international exchange or knowledge and skills is beyond the personal budget of most individuals, scholarship provision helps to fill the gap. Typically a three-way partnership operates: finances come from the scholarship provider, an employer grants paid leave of absence, and much time, energy, enthusiasm and professional expertise are invested by the travel scholar before, during and after the study visit.

TRAVEL SCHOLARSHIP ADVERTISING

Because of the dynamic and diverse nature of scholarship availability, general comment on, rather than detailed discussion of, the various types follows. Different groups and grades of staff often have access to a variety of scholarships at different points in a career. There are some general guidelines, however, which will increase awareness of scholarship availability.

Local scholarships

These are open to staff working in a specific hospital, city or region, for example, and are often only advertised locally. They may be open to one professional group, or to all health care professions. Typically, information is circulated via the line management structure, is posted on notice boards, or is circulated by the local branch of a professional organization.

Professional journals

Professional journals are an excellent source of scholarship information available on a national basis. The advertisement might be a formal one inviting applications, or form part of a news item. Looking at back copies of a number of professional journals will give a feel for where information tends to be published. Some scholarships are multi-disciplinary; others are international in their eligibility. It is therefore important to scan journals of other health care disciplines published in this country and abroad.

The publications of trade unions and professional organizations often include information regarding scholarships. Being a member of one or more of these bodies ensures access to their publications, and further material can be obtained from libraries.

The general press

Some scholarships are advertised in the general press. These are usually available to the general public as well as to health care professionals. For example a major scholarship provider in the United Kingdom offers a number of scholarships annually and specifies a range of subject categories. The categories might include ones not specific to health care professions, horse training, and ship's carpentry, for example. Other subjects, however, may relate specifically to health care, for example self-medication in the elderly, health education, and alternative medicine.

When considering applying for a scholarship, the application requirements contained in the advertisement must be studied and/or any additional information must be requested. It is necessary to consider whether, in the written application, the sponsors can be convinced that undertaking a foreign study tour is appropriate at this stage of a career. This can be done by ensuring that the CV clearly demonstrates that local and national opportunities have been exhausted. The application will be strengthened if it is easy to understand. Although some handwriting may be relatively easy to read, it can be tiring or difficult to read for a long period.

WRITING THE APPLICATION

The possibility of a successful application can be increased by considering the following. Sponsors will expect to be provided with written evidence of active professional commitment and involvement. The applicant must be prepared to provide evidence of being a specialist in the subject area; of familiarity with and/or having contributed to the subject literature; and of an awareness of local and national centres of excellence. Referees must be able to confirm an applicant's subject expertise, and that he or she has the ability to make good use of the experience.

Where possible, the applicant should provide written confirmation from potential study tour hosts that appropriate experiences can be provided by them. This will enhance the application and improve the possibility of success. Potential hosts must be identified and contacted well in advance of the scholarship application. Most are generally willing to enter into a tentative arrangement for a visit should the application prove successful. Contact with potential hosts can be made personally, with or without assistance from a professional organization. Funding organizations use a variety of application forms for would-be travel scholars. Usually, they request information such as:

Curriculum vitae or résumé
The names and addresses of two referees
Details of the visit (place(s), duration, etc.)
Purpose of the visit
Supporting material
Estimates of costs (possibly)

Curriculum vitae or résumé

The inclusion of a curriculum vitae, or a résumé if that is what is requested, places the application in the context of previous professional training, experience and development. The CV will demonstrate that the visit is an extension of previous professional activity. The more professionally involved and productive the applicant, as demonstrated by the content of a CV, the greater the possibility of success. (See Chapter 16, 'Curriculum Vitae and Résumé').

Referees

Referees are usually asked to support the application, comment on its relevance to the applicant's specialist area, and confirm details of experience and general suitability. As with all referees, they must be *asked* to provide a reference and if they agree must be given a copy of the application, all supporting papers, and a CV. Some organizations only contact shortlisted candidates' referees; others contact all referees.

Details of the visit

Successful applications can range from the vague, 'To visit four well known post-amputation rehabilitation units in Australia', for example, to the very specific: 'To visit units A, B, C and D . . .'. The more specific the plans are, the better. Applicants will be asked to indicate the length of the visit and the anticipated starting date.

Most funding bodies do not regard the visit plan as being totally inflexible. It may, for example, be necessary to alter the dates or make adjustments to the itinerary for any of a number of reasons. However, within this flexible framework it is usually difficult to make major changes such as altering the purpose of the visit.

Purpose of the visit

Scholarship sources obviously wish to ensure that they support applicants who will use the visit to make a substantial contribution to their personal and professional development and to the work of their profession or a specialist part of it. The sponsor has to be convinced that the visit will help improve the applicant's professional contribution and that of colleagues with whom the experience will be shared by way of talks and publications.

Supporting material

Although some funding bodies specifically request that no enclosures accompany the application form, others welcome additional relevant material. This might include:

A curriculum vitae
Letter of support from employer
Letters from places to be visited
Evidence to support choice of places to be visited, with reference to
  appropriate publications of their staff.

Estimate of costs

It is usual for sponsoring bodies to ask for at least an estimate of the overall cost of the proposed study tour. Alternatively, a detailed estimate of the component parts of the overall costs may be requested. In either case, the following list of items can be costed to produce either an overall or detailed estimate. These are examples only: not all items will be included in all applications.

Travel, international and between places to be visited
Local travel (bus, taxi, etc.)
Travel insurance
Accommodation
Meals
Postage, telephone, stationery, photocopying
Handheld dictating machine
Professional literature
Interpreter
Report preparation, secretary

THE INTERVIEW

Funding organizations usually interview a small number of shortlisted applicants. The choice is strongly influenced by the quality of the written material forming and supporting the application. A purpose of the interview is to discuss the content of the application form and supporting material, to deal with issues not covered in them, and to enable interviewers to examine applicants' professional and personal backgrounds. Applicants should expect to be asked to elaborate on any aspect of the materials submitted. For example, if it is claimed that a formal literature review of the subject of the proposed study tour has recently been undertaken, he or she should be prepared to discuss specific examples. If the application form states that Unit Y is a centre of excellence, it may be necessary to justify that claim.

Interviewees will probably be asked to describe how they will share the experience with colleagues: by publishing a report in the professional press, for example. They must be prepared to discuss where, when and how a study tour report might be published and otherwise made available. Interview questions may also focus on how change might be initiated after the visit. It is impossible to predict the questions that might be asked in this type of interview. However, if the application is well prepared and is fully supported by additional material such as a well written CV, the possibility of success is increased.

Interview outcome

In due course applicants are informed of the outcome of the interview. Success is easy to accept; failure less so. The fear of failure may prevent some potentially successful applicants from applying. However, it is worth remembering that, for each successful applicant, there are many equally suitable ones who do not succeed. It should also be borne in mind that success might come with a second, fourth or seventh attempt. Failure *might* mean that the awarding body feels that the proposal should not be supported. More often, it results from limitations on scholarship finances, some good applications being refused because of limited funds. The unsuccessful applicant should take a critical look at the application and discuss it with the referees. Perhaps it might be improved for a future application, or it might be possible to use it on future occasions in an unchanged form. In either event, if potential hosts have already been contacted, it is important to get in touch with them again and request permission to continue to use their letters of support in future applications.

ARRANGING THE STUDY TOUR

If the application is successful, much has to be done in planning the study tour. It is normal to get details of the amount of the scholarship award at this stage, and *possibly* a request to submit details of expenditure after the visit. Full funds might be sent on a specified date, or the organization may arrange to pay major travel costs to a travel agent and send the balance nearer the start of the tour. Queries regarding financial arrangements can easily be answered by contacting the sponsors.

After accepting the award, written advice on how to plan the tour may be provided. Some funding bodies provide excellent information developed from years of experience; others provide very little. Professional bodies often have an overseas department willing to provide advice on many aspects of planning and undertaking a study tour. It is best to contact such an organization as soon as possible and ask if it provides this service.

It will be necessary to discuss the visit with an employer or immediate line manager and confirm the previous provisional request for leave of absence if this is necessary. Next, firm dates for the tour must be set and overseas hosts must be notified. If tentative arrangements have been made earlier, confirming these will not present problems. If not, potential hosts must be contacted immediately, enclosing full personal details, an explanation of the objectives of the visit and of the nature of the scholarship, and a full CV. They must be provided with the name of the funding organization and, where appropriate, any special conditions attached to the award. Giving full details at this stage will avoid delay in receiving a clear reply to the request to visit, and prevent inappropriate arrangements being made. Later, a specific timetable for the visit and accommodation requirements must be discussed and advice sought regarding internal travel if more than one place is to be visited. It is also important to consider whether or not the services of an interpreter need to be purchased or otherwise obtained.

Various routine personal arrangements have to be made for being away from home. These can range from cancelling the milk delivery to having the cat taken care of. Travel insurance must be arranged, validity of a passport must be checked and visas obtained where necessary. Other arrangements that must be made include those for carrying and/or transferring funds and for international and major domestic travel. The necessary clothing must be packed and any health checks and immunizations must be carried out. Travel details are best discussed with a travel agent and the organization being visited.

Hosts may extend an invitation to the travel scholar to talk about the subject of the visit as a result of formal or informal contact with colleagues in the host institution(s). They might also request a more general talk on aspects of health care and professional education in the travel scholar's country. Ideally, the hosts should have made these requests before departure, but this may not have been possible, they may simply have been overlooked, or they may have been made as a polite afterthought. In any event it may be prudent to take some written notes regarding personal work, the health care system generally, professional education and so on. These might not be needed, but will enable a formal or informal talk to be given at short notice.

The time required to finalize the arrangements will depend on a number of things, including whether or not firm contacts with potential hosts have already been made. Visits to some countries, the USA and Western Europe for example, can often be arranged quickly and relatively informally. Visits to some other countries such as those in Eastern Europe have, until recently, taken very much longer. Some time ago I spent six months planning a study visit to Poland. Some of the positive formal replies from hosts arrived days before the start of the visit; others reached this country after my arrival in Poland. All planning should therefore be done as far as possible in advance of the visit.

THE VISIT

In addition to providing those experiences which will meet the specific objectives of the visit, hosts might identify additional ones which, although not central to it, are related to it or to the scholar's general professional background. After arrival it is not unusual to be told of an additional person or place in the area which may be of interest. It is therefore important to ensure that the timetable is sufficiently flexible to make such an additional visit possible.

As well as the inevitable culture shock, possibly made worse by jet lag, considerable sensory overload may be experienced by the travel scholar as a result of exposure to new information and experiences. This is made worse if visiting many centres for short periods of time, rather than making fewer, longer visits. The following hints will increase the value of the visit.

- The travel scholar should arrive at the first destination in time to allow a few days' rest before starting to visit the hosts. This is particularly important if the country's culture differs substantially from the scholar's own.
- It is advisable to visit a few, rather than many, different locations in the country/countries; one week is a reasonable minimum period for each.
- The timetable should include enough time for rest, reflection, note taking and social activity.

The travel scholar should expect to encounter a large amount of new experiences and information; it is therefore important to consider how these will be recorded. Unless decisions are made regarding this before the visit, there is a risk of it being done badly and much being forgotten before the tour ends. Some note taking will be possible: during meetings with individuals or small groups, for example. However, there is the possibility that taking notes will disrupt or slow down information exchange. Alternatively, notes may be prepared at the end of each day, or at the end of each meeting during the day, depending on the time available between meetings and visits. Using a handheld micro-recorder is one means of note taking, enabling the recording of notes at the end of each day or, if the timetable permits, during the day between visits and meetings. It is important to collect relevant documents, policy statements, care plans, publications and handouts of various forms from each of the places visited. These can be used as an aid to subsequent report writing or can be included as appendices. If such documents exist but are not available during the visit, it is advisable to ask that they be sent to you; they are invaluable.

WRITING THE REPORT

One outcome of all study tours is writing the inevitable, necessary and occasionally difficult report for the sponsors and for publication. Writing a formal report is a condition of virtually all scholarship awards. It is also an important means of sharing the experience with others. The report might be structured in one of a number of ways including the chronological one (starting with the first place visited and ending with the last) or be arranged by subject. In the latter approach, the material must be examined and different topics described and identified irrespective of the point in the visit at which the experience was provided. Examples might include health education, in-service training, multidisciplinary case conferences, research funding and specialist libraries, all relating to a particular discipline or specialty.

There is no blueprint to guarantee success when writing a study tour report. Success will be determined by the content of the notes and other information collected during the visit. It is also influenced by reading reports written by previous travel scholars funded by the sponsoring organization. Example 44 demonstrates a possible report structure.

Example 44

Travel scholarship report structure

Personal details
Details of the scholarship awarding body
Clinical/academic details of the host establishment(s)
The reasons for undertaking the visit
How this was achieved
Where and when the visit took place
A description of information collected during the visit
Interpretation of the information collected
Applicability of the information to the profession and to health care
    generally
Formal acknowledgement of the sponsor and host(s)

The report must be written with a sensitivity and understanding that take account of the differing values and histories of the places visited and of the brevity of the visit. The temptation to be overcritical of other systems can be overcome by recognizing the limitations of the visit, and by learning from it rather than by making generalized statements based on limited experience.

SHARING THE EXPERIENCE

When the report is complete, it can be adapted for publication in a professional journal. It can be shortened to form an article, or discrete parts can be selected to form more than one article. Opportunities should be sought to inform colleagues of the visit by making a copy of the report available to them, and by speaking at seminars, study days and conferences. In addition to submitting the report to the sponsor a full copy should be sent to the overseas hosts, and one should also be placed in the staff library.

Chapter 15 (Articles) can be used to provide a structure for the study tour report and for the article(s) that develop from it.

Chapter 21
Writing Technology

In today's technological world there seem to be aids that can assist with almost every task that once was labour intensive. Not very long ago the budding writer would spend many hours, days or even months planning, drafting and polishing a piece of work prior to having it typed ready for sharing with a wider audience. Today most writers can, if they wish, capture their earliest thoughts, develop their ideas, produce high quality printed early drafts for comment, then with final editing create a tight, well structured text all at a fraction of the cost with the aid of a word processor.

It is not the intention of this chapter to recommend any one type of word processor or indeed advise on the supporting equipment that will need to be purchased. The purpose of this chapter is to identify the options available and the features that writing technology can offer.

HARDWARE

Hardware is the term used for the equipment. It is analogous to the ink, pen and paper used by a traditional author. There are many different types of hardware that can be used to support writing. However, all in essence can be traced back to or are associated with developments of either the standard typewriter or the personal computer, both of which have evolved to produce systems that will enable processing of the written word in a flexible, efficient and cost-effective way.

Dedicated word processors

Systems that have evolved from a standard typewriter are often referred to as dedicated word processors. Over a number of years more and more features have been added.

Electric typewriters were the first stage of development. The incorporation of electromechanical components in a standard typewriter brought considerable benefits to the would-be writer. Using a manual machine, a proficient typist can produce excellent copy that has characters of equal darkness and correct alignment. Unfortunately, not all professionals are so proficient with manual machines. The advent of electric typewriters allowed all writers, with practice, to produce text comparable to that generated by an excellent typist. Most of these machines still use a standard inked ribbon but often in addition have a white ribbon that overtypes errors so that any correction can be typed in on top. Provided that white paper is used, errors are seldom seen. However, if paper other than white is preferred, any corrected text becomes visible to the reader. Electric typewriters can still be purchased but most manufacturers are phasing out this type of machine in favour of electronic models.

As technology has advanced, electromechanical components have tended to be replaced by electronic systems. Instead of having many typewriter keys that have to travel individually and strike the page, an electronic typewriter has a single rotating wheel with all the characters upon it. The wheel then moves along the carriage and the appropriate character is struck. In one single step the vast majority of moving parts have been removed from the machine. This had several advantages. The electronic typewriter is far more reliable. The machine is much more portable since its weight is greatly reduced. Most machines accept interchangeable character wheels, which enable the writer to change the style of print as well as the size. In addition, electronic typewriters tend to use a special type of ribbon. This means that if an error is made it can be lifted off the paper. Once corrected, errors are almost entirely invisible to the average reader even if coloured paper is used. A trip down to the local high street supplier of office equipment will reveal a wide selection of electronic typewriters, many of which will have additional features.

Some electronic typewriters can store work before actually typing it on to a page of paper. In some cases, this memory feature is an integral part of the machine; in others, work can be stored on a floppy disk. Floppy disks can be thought of as a recording medium that stores work in an electronic format which can be retrieved later. This facility offers the opportunity to store and then edit text in a far more flexible manner. There is no need to retype an entire paper; the article can simply be retrieved and those parts that require amendment changed. The machine is then made ready to type another revised copy. The more advanced models of electronic typewriter will also offer some of the features of a fully dedicated word processor, such as automatic justification (ensuring that both left and right margins are parallel to one another), spell checking, and cut and paste editing (a way of moving text about the page without having to retype it).

Dedicated word processors are the point on the evolutionary ladder at which personal computers and manual typewriters merged. These dedicated machines have a wide variety of features which assist in the manipulation of text and graphics. In hardware terms they look almost identical to a personal computer. However, in some cases the machine will have an integral screen, keyboard and printer. The software, a computer program, which in the case of a dedicated word processor is the part of the machine that allows a writer to manipulate the text, is usually stored on a silicon chip and is available as soon as the machine is switched on. The software has usually been specially written for the machine and hence often has a non-standard instruction set (the rules and special keys that have to be pressed or followed to manipulate text). Dedicated word processors are often less expensive than a personal computer but are less flexible. By definition they can only word process. This may not be a problem if manipulating text is all that is required. However, if graphics, bar charts, pie charts, pictures or diagrams are to be integrated, this limitation of the dedicated word processor may cause problems.

Personal computers as word processors

First and foremost a personal computer is a computer! This seems obvious but it is this feature that provides the greatest flexibility and cause for confusion.

Personal computers can run many different types of software, not just word processing packages, but spreadsheets, databases, graphics, and statistics packages to name only a few. Indeed it is possible to buy integrated packages which allow a user to access all these applications seemingly almost all at once.

When using a personal computer for the purposes of word processing, it is the software, the word processing package, that controls the way text is manipulated. Many different software packages can be used, all offering a variation of the standard word processor on the same personal computer. Therefore, if a particular package does not meet all the writer's needs, it should be possible to buy another that does.

Personal computers can also support various pieces of specialist hardware in addition to a wide variety of printers.

Printers

Any writer considering using a personal computer to assist in the production of a piece of work must consider the quality of print that the final document will give to potential readers. If the writer is hoping to have the work published, initial impressions are important and due consideration must be given to the selection of an appropriate printer.

Four different types of printer are commonly available. Each has specific advantages and disadvantages but in essence it is the main use to be made of the printer, the desired quality of print and the amount of money available that should determine the choice.

Laser printers

Laser printers are considered by many writers to be the best in terms of print quality but are also the most expensive. They are able to produce both high quality text and graphics. They work on the same principle as a photocopier and hence use cartridges of 'toner' rather than ink. These cartridges can be quite expensive but are relatively long lasting. Thus, if considering the purchase of such a machine, it is important to enquire about the cost and availability of such consumables. Laser printers can produce text at a rate of several pages per minute which is 'copy ready', that is, ready for input into a publisher's typesetting system (more details of this are given in the next section). Recently, colour laser printers have come on to the market but the cost for most people is prohibitive unless high volumes of material, probably on a commercial basis, are to be produced.

Ink jet printers

Ink jet printers, sometimes referred to as paint jet machines, have increased in popularity as their costs have come into line with those of dot matrix impact printers. The quality produced is very high and in some cases as good as the output of laser printers. As the name suggests, ink jet printers work by spraying ink on to the paper. Unfortunately, if the room in which work is being printed is cold and/or damp, the ink may take a minute or two to dry and hence may smudge – a rare problem but one worth mentioning. Like laser printers, ink jet printers are silent, can produce flexible print in a variety of styles (fonts), and can deal easily with graphs or other diagrams. Ink jet printers put colour printing into the price range of most writers and can be particularly useful if graphs or pie charts are to be integrated into the text.

Dot matrix printers

Dot matrix printers are perhaps the most readily available type of printer that can be used to produce hard copy. In recent years print quality has improved considerably and in some cases the material produced is almost as good as the output of other types of printer. Dot matrix printers can produce both text and graphic output. They do this by striking a ribbon of ink against the paper with a number of small pins to produce dots. There are two standards of printer commonly available, 9-pin or 24-pin. The latter produces better quality output since the dots are closer together. Most dot matrix printers can produce print in either a draft or near letter quality (NLQ) form. Draft format is much quicker and perfectly acceptable for early working copies of documents, but NLQ standard should be used before submitting the final paper for publication. One word of caution, if noise is an issue: dot matrix machines are far from silent, especially if using NLQ mode.

Daisy wheel printers

Daisy wheel printers produce high quality print but are less flexible than the other types of printer since they cannot deal with graphical or diagram output. These printers allow the use of interchangeable wheels which can offer a selection of typefaces and size of print. However, since it is necessary to physically change the wheel it is not possible to readily mix and match styles or sizes on a single page. Like dot matrix printers, daisy wheel machines are noisy and tend to be slow. The costs of daisy wheel printers are comparable to those of ink jet and dot matrix machines. Nowadays, owing to their lack of popularity and flexibility, they are more difficult to obtain. If planning to make a once and for all purchase, it should be borne in mind that consumables and spare parts may be difficult to obtain a few years later.

Specialist hardware

Personal computers support a number of specialist pieces of hardware that can significantly ease the writing process.

Mice

For those writers who do not get text word perfect first time, mice are a useful addition that can ease the editing process. A mouse is simply a small, oblong 50 × 100 mm (2 in × 4 in) pointing device with two or three buttons that is connected to the computer by means of a cable. The mouse allows text to be marked on the screen, removed all together or shifted to another part of the document. It can also be used to set up the layout of pages and to speed up the process of issuing commands to the word processing package.

Scanners

Scanners are useful if there is a need to incorporate an existing diagram or photograph into a paper. They work on the same principle as a facsimile machine, converting the image, line by line, into a signal that can then be processed and incorporated into a document. Two types of scanner are available: handheld, which look like an inverted letter T; and flat-bed machines, which are similar to a small photocopier. Scanners can be extremely useful for enabling writers to add graphics or diagrammatic material, but care must be taken not to infringe the copyright of the original author.

SOFTWARE PACKAGES

There are a number of packages that can assist in the development of professional writing skills. If a personal computer is selected as opposed to a dedicated system, it will be necessary to purchase a word processing package that will, along with appropriate hardware, facilitate the production of the text. Other packages, such as databases, spreadsheets and statistics and graphics software, can be used to complement the system, but the central purchase should be an appropriate word processor.

Word processors

Word processors can vary considerably both in their cost and in their complexity. It is not the intention of this chapter to teach a potential user how to use a word processor. However, features that should influence the choice in purchasing any system will be identified. When considering the purchase or use of a word processor, the availability of ready advice is an important point to consider. If colleagues are well versed in the use of a particular package, their views should be sought. Selecting a well known package may be the best solution for those unfamiliar with the vast array of packages now available.

Controlling word processors

There are three main ways of controlling the commands that a word processor can offer: function keys, pull-down menus, or keystroke combinations.

All computer keyboards have several, usually 12, function keys located along the top or along the left- or right-hand sides of the keyboard and numbered from F1 to F12. By pressing the various function keys, either on their own or in conjunction with the 'SHIFT', 'CTRL' or 'ALT' keys, the various word processor commands can be used.

Pull-down menus can be accessed by highlighting a menu bar at the top of the screen. This can be done by means of a mouse or by pressing a special keystroke combination. For example, pressing 'ALT' and 'F' simultaneously may access the pull-down menu on file handling. If a system that offers pull-down menus is purchased, a mouse should be considered an essential addition to the machine. Without a mouse it is difficult to take full advantage of the flexibility that pull-down menus offer.

Although keystroke combinations were common in the earlier generation of word processing packages and are still available as an alternative, to a certain extent they have gone out of favour. The main difficulty with using keystroke combinations is that users need to remember them or look them up. For a proficient typist who uses the system regularly, recalling keystroke combinations may not be a problem. However, most people find the use of function keys or pull-down menus much more user friendly.

File handling

When writing a paper using a word processor, it will be necessary to save the completed document so that it can be retrieved and edited, amended or appended later. Sometimes writers may wish to save a file in a format that can be read by another system – to send the material to a publisher, a teacher or a friend. If no other option is available, material can be stored in ASCII (American Standard Code for Information Interchange) format since this is normally readable on other systems. However, instructions in one format (requesting the use of bold type, for example) may be lost if a file is stored in ASCII. Thus, at the very least, the intending user must make sure that any package can both read and write in this format. More sophisticated systems will offer the choice of being able to read and write files in all the common word processing formats, for example WordPerfect, WordStar, and Microsoft Word.

On-screen help

The better word processing packages will offer on screen help. This will allow writers to ask for clues or an explanation on how to use a specific command or action. The more advanced systems even allow for different levels of help. More advanced users can even disable the function if confident that it will not be required.

Spell checker

A very useful feature which most word processors offer is a spelling checker. This can check the spelling of words individually, in sections of the document or throughout the entire file. Today's spell-checking systems will identify mistakes and offer a suggestion which is the system's best guess at what the correct spelling of the word should be. However, the use of a spell checker does not identify errors in grammar or typographical errors which happen to result in the correct spelling of a word. For example, if, instead of 'word', 'ward' had been typed, a spell checker would not pick up the error. The moral of this for an aspiring writer is not to rely on a spell checker for proofreading.

A common problem that may be encountered by those new to the purchase of writing technology is that a spell checker that uses American rather than British spelling may be included with the word processor. Most word processors now offer a choice but it is important to be careful to get the appropriate version. In a specialist field many words may be used that do not appear in the standard spell-checking dictionary. It is therefore essential that any package offers the option to add words so as to customize the dictionary as necessary.

Some packages can also use foreign language versions as an add-on option. This can be useful if material is likely to be published in non-English journals.

Thesaurus

Some of the basic word-processing packages do not offer a thesaurus whereas most of the more advanced systems include one as standard. A good thesaurus will offer a meaning, synonyms and antonyms.

Grammar checking

Some of the most advanced packages offer a grammar checking facility. This will analyse writing and apply rules of grammar to diagnose whether there are any errors. Often suggestions on how to improve the text will be made, and on completion of the analysis of the document feedback on the readability of the paper is given. The readability index may be derived via one of a number of approaches, but in essence it is calculated on the basis of sentence and paragraph length and sentence construction.

Page preview

A page preview facility will allow writers to see on the screen how the written paper will appear, page by page, on paper. This can be very useful since it enables the writer to get an impression of the appearance of the text without having to print out the document. This is often referred to as the WYSIWYG feature (What You See Is What You Get). It can be particularly valuable if there is a need to insert graphs or diagrams throughout the text.

Edit functions

The real power of a word processor is in the system's ability to edit text. Single characters, words, sentences, paragraphs or even whole chapters can be readily inserted, deleted or moved. The editing process does not introduce errors into parts of the text which are left unaltered. Traditionally, having a manuscript retyped often led to the introduction of new errors in previously correct parts of the text.

If a writer examines a paper and decides that a paragraph or section is out of order and needs to be moved to another part of the document, this can be done easily. The text is simply highlighted, then moved to the new position in the paper.

Sometimes writers may decide to find and replace a certain word throughout the document so as to enable a paper to be adjusted to the house style of a certain journal. For example if a paper is to be published in a medically oriented journal, the term 'patient' could be used, but if it is to be submitted to a social science publication it might be more appropriate to replace 'patient' with 'client'. This can be done automatically if a FIND and REPLACE edit function is available.

Insertion of graphs, diagrams or pictures

Sophisticated word processing packages will allow writers to insert into the body of the text any graphical, diagrammatic or photographic figures. These can then be printed out as an integral part of the text rather than having to cut and physically paste them in later. Some packages allow insertions to be prepared in another piece of software such as a graphics package, then transferred into the word processor. Others require the use of a scanner to prepare material for insertion.

Layout and format commands

If papers or documents are written for a number of journals, it is likely that work will need to be presented using slightly different layouts. For example, the print margins, left, right, top and bottom may need to be altered or the line spacing and justification requirements may differ. All these requirements can be dealt with easily, and any document can be edited using the appropriate layout and format commands to meet the requirements of any publisher. Therefore if a paper is written with one journal in mind but subsequently it is decided to submit it to another, the document can easily be restructured without having to retype it.

Other software packages

There are a number of additional applications packages that can be used effectively by a writer. Applications such as databases, spreadsheets and statistical analysis, or graphics packages can all be used either independently of the word processor or as a comprehensive integrated package that offers a variety of functions and facilities.

Databases

Databases can be of considerable value to the budding author since they can store references accurately in a readily accessible format. With a little practice it is possible to get a database containing references to print out its contents in such a way as to meet the requirements of most journals. This can then be inserted in the appropriate section of the paper without having to retype the material.

If a writer conducts original research, a database can be a useful tool for storing data that can then be interrogated (sorted and queried) and analysed. Most commercial databases will offer a minimum of descriptive statistical functions. For more advanced analysis a specific statistical package may be required. Some databases will allow data to be sent or transferred to statistical packages relatively easily; others can make life difficult. If this feature is a possible requirement, the supplier should be questioned carefully.

Statistical analysis packages

Statistical analysis packages are now readily available for most personal computers and can perform basic and advanced analysis with relative ease. Many statistical packages can present data automatically in a well laid out format that can be edited (cut and pasted) straight into a paper.

Statistical packages can be expensive and do take up large amounts of disk space. In addition, if they are used frequently for analyses that are calculation intensive, it may be necessary to increase the computational capacity of the computer by adding extra components such as a maths co-processor (a type of silicon chip designed specifically for carrying out mathematical calculations).

Graphics packages

Graphics packages, as the name suggests, can produce graphical output in a variety of formats. Thus bar charts, histograms, pie charts and scattergrams should all be readily available. Data for the graphs can be entered directly into the package manually or automatically from a database, a statistics package or a spreadsheet. The data can then be displayed using any of the example formats above, and edited, by changing scales or layout, to maximize visual impact. The more sophisticated graphics packages will allow the finished figure to be exported (transferred) straight into the word processor or into a format that can produce slides or acetates for presentations.

Spreadsheets

Spreadsheets can be thought of as a giant matrix which can be asked to carry out various mathematical calculations. They are frequently used when people wish to carry out modelling or 'what if' calculations. Spreadsheets often have in-built capabilities that will allow the generation of all standard forms of graphs. Again an advanced system will have a feature that can enable material to be transferred directly to a word processing package.

CONCLUSIONS

The purpose of this chapter was to explain some of the advantages that can be obtained from using writing technology. Various writing tools can be used to assist in the production and publication of work. Although every word processor tends to be a little different from most others, time taken to master one package will develop skills that are readily transferable to other systems.

Although publishers still accept hard copy, many will ask for and prefer writers to submit manuscripts in electronic format. This speeds up the publishing process since there is no need to retype the paper and in some cases the document can be passed electronically to a type-setting machine. This has the advantage of limiting the risk of introducing new errors since there is no need to have someone type the paper again. An interim stage that some publishers are now using is that of document scanning. This is where a document can be scanned from the hard copy into a computer and then edited ready for publishing. If a publisher uses document scanning, it is essential that a good clear hard copy which can then be electronically read is provided.

Writing technology can make a writer's life much easier. It can allow the writer to draft and re-draft a document with great ease. It can check spelling and grammar and even offer alternatives for those words that seem to be being used too often. However, technology can only facilitate the process: It cannot provide inspiration, for technology is but a tool to be used.

Chapter 22
Economics of Writing

Some health care staff find the subject of money as it relates to writing for a professional readership embarrassing, if not unpalatable. Recently a colleague said, rather apologetically, during a discussion of professional writing opportunities, 'I know this isn't a very professional question, but do writers get paid for their work?' Apart from indicating a naiveté about the economics of writing, the question is indicative of the commonly held view that professionalism, as it relates to writing for publication, and money are incompatible. The reply to that question included a discussion of the extent to which writers get paid and a clear indication that such payment was reasonable, indeed essential. There can be little doubt that writers from the health care professions, particularly those who write for publication, need to be *very* aware of the economics of writing.

Almost all writing endeavours involve financial cost to the writer, occasionally income and perhaps profit, and possibly the payment of income tax. In some though not all instances, the income derived from writing may partly or wholly offset costs. However, as soon as income is received, it becomes a subject of interest to the collectors of income tax.

Three related topics are dealt with in this chapter: writing costs, income from writing, and income tax. The discussion is not comprehensive but it will draw attention to a number of financial issues and increase awareness of the whole question of the economics of writing. Similarly, the discussion will *not* constitute an income tax guide. Anyone in doubt about any financial points, particularly in relation to income tax, is advised to consult an accountant. The chapter's contents relate to taxation regulations in the UK; readers from elsewhere should consult advisors in their own countries.

Whilst health care professionals are unlikely to get rich by writing for publications, it is as well to keep expenditure to a minimum, to maximize income, and keep tax bills to a (legal) minimum. By so doing, the possibility of making a net loss is decreased and that of making a modest profit is increased. Although most of those with whom the writer comes into contact, including publishers, are anxious to give a 'fair deal' and to receive value for money, it is as well for the beginner to know some of the ground rules.

WRITING COSTS

The costs of writing are often composed of a number of apparently small sums of money. Each outlay may in itself seem minimal; the total cost, however, might be quite considerable and should be taken into account by those who become involved in writing for publication.

The items of expenditure covered in this section relate to the range of writing activities discussed in this book. Some items, typing for example, relate to almost all kinds of work whereas others, such as indexing, relate only to writing a book. It is therefore necessary for the reader to be selective in the application of the material, remembering that not all items will apply to all types of writing.

With few exceptions, and then mainly for illustrative purposes, actual costs will not be included for two reasons. First they will obviously vary from place to place and may depend on shopping around for the best buy. Secondly, costs change over time, resulting in any amounts stated quickly going out of date. The main purpose here is to show the type and variety of costs rather than to describe what these might actually be.

Most of this section involves income tax implications, the difference between approved expenditure and income being the amounts on which income tax is paid – assuming of course that the recipient is a tax payer. For this reason it is essential that accurate records be kept of all income and expenditure. When possible, *receipts* or any other proof of expenditure must be obtained and kept. These records, which must be retained for some years after the event, will only be used if items of expenditure are challenged by the income tax authorities. In addition to fulfilling taxation requirements, consideration of all writing costs will enable a personal budget to be worked out and in relation to consultancy work will help to determine a reasonable charge for the work.

For income tax purposes some items of expenditure, that is those which are purchased and used exclusively for writing for publication, can be included in full: the cost of posting a manuscript to a publisher, for example. Other items, that is those which are not purchased and used exclusively for writing for publication, are included on a pro rata basis. For example, if a word processor is bought for professional writing purposes *and* for family use, a judgement has to be made as to the proportion of its use, 50% for example, for writing activities. Thus, half of the cost of the word processor, disks, typing ribbons, maintenance and so on would be counted as expenditure for tax purposes. After each of the examples of items of expenditure below, there appears a guide as to whether the item is likely to be regarded on a 'pro rata' or 'in full' basis. This is a decision that can only be made by the writer, and is one that may or may not be accepted by the income tax staff.

Writing materials

A good supply of lined and unlined notepaper, pencils, pens and erasers are the minimum tools for the beginner. Sticky tape, paperclips and scissors are useful for the frequent cutting and pasting necessary when work enters its various draft forms. These basic materials are obvious examples of costs which, in themselves, are rather insignificant. However, in addition to other expenditure they become increasingly large. (*In full.*)

Postage and telephone

Communication costs can be considerable, particularly where frequent contact has to be made with co-writers of a book or article. Postage costs are relatively easy to record since receipts can be obtained for postage stamps and other postal costs. Unless itemized telephone bills can be obtained, telephone costs are rather more difficult to record. However a brief note of the recipient of each call, along with an estimate of cost, should suffice. It is important to record postage and telephone costs arising from contact with a publisher and from 'researching' the subject. The cost of stationery, packaging materials and *all* other costs of communicating with others must be recorded. (*In full.*)

Typing

Although the availability of word processors makes it possible for writers to become good amateur typists, many will have neither the time nor the inclination and will prefer to hire a professional secretary. Many secretaries will type the manuscripts of articles, books and other items for publication in their spare time; alternatively, a typing/secretarial agency may be used. Charges will be either by the hour or by the page. Payment per page, rather than by the hour, makes budgeting and cost containment much easier. Also, it does not matter whether the typist produces six or sixteen pages per hour. It is best to get a few quotations, particularly for longer pieces of work, in order to establish the best buy and to establish the normal cost range. A clear agreement regarding typing specifications and cost must be made *before* the work begins. Items to be negotiated whoever is doing the typing include the following. Does the cost per page include the production of copies? What is the type spacing to be used, for example single or double? Does the cost cover correction of typist errors? (It should.) How will writer errors and corrections be paid for? Will a word processor be used? (It is preferable that one be used.) What is the timescale for completion including corrections?

If the work is being done by a person or an agency not used before, it is advisable to ask for a two- or three-page sample of work before a formal agreement is reached. A copy of the bill and receipt of payment must be stored for future use. (*In full.*)

Artwork and photography

If photographs or art illustrations such as line drawings are required, publishers should be asked if they can provide these services either free or at a cost. For example, some publishers have a library of photographs or have a resident graphic artist who can produce line drawings according to a writer's specifications. Alternatively assistance might be available, at a cost, from a place of work, from the graphics department of a college or university or, increasingly commonly, from a range of shops selling art, photographic and graphic assistance to the general public.

If the publication is to include photographs, it might be best to employ a professional photographer. If so, it is important to ask for a quotation, and only to pay for a professional job. As with other costs, the receipt must be retained.

Work such as line drawings may be done by a graphic artist on the basis of a payment for each drawing. Requirements must be discussed with the artist and a single 'sample' commissioned before making further arrangements. (*In full.*)

Professional books and journals

All textbooks, including a dictionary, thesaurus and other professional reference books, are part of the cost of writing. This is particularly so when a textbook or a number of articles are being written. Regular purchase of professional journals, or a subscription to one or more, can also be included even though not all issues will contain material of particular relevance to the research being undertaken in relation to current writing activities. (*In full or pro rata.*)

Travel

Travel, whether it be to collect material for publication or to discuss work with the publisher or other contributors to the book or article, can add considerably to writing costs. This also applies to additional living and subsistence costs, for example meals and hotel bills, incurred during travel. Two means of calculating actual travel costs can be used: public transport cost or reasonable and recognized rate per mile travelled. For the former, receipts should be obtained; the latter requires a personal record of mileage travelled. Both require records of the date and purpose of the journey. (*In full.*)

Professional fees

If the services of an accountant are used and paid for in relation to preparing accounts for income tax purposes, the fee can be set against income for tax purposes. The same point applies if a lawyer is consulted in relation to a contract for example, and if the services of a literary agent, professional indexer, artist or photographer are used. (*In full.*)

Assistant's fees

If another person such as a professional colleague is paid a fee for work done on a manuscript, reviewing one or more drafts for example, this is regarded as expenditure for taxation purposes. (*In full.*)

Rent, mortgage, heating, lighting

If the writing is done at home, particularly if it is a substantial amount such as a book, part of the cost of heating, lighting, air conditioning and rent or mortgage should be regarded as writing costs. The exact amount of these costs (as a proportion of the actual cost of these items) which can be offset against taxation of future income from the published work should be discussed directly with the income tax authorities, or with an accountant. (*Pro rata.*)

Indexing

Many publishers will, if required, provide the name(s) of professional indexer(s) who will prepare a book index. This contact may be direct but more usually is made via the society to which professional indexers belong. Indexing charges may be based on the length of the manuscript and/or the length of the index. (*In full.*)

Equipment purchase, repair and replacement

Equipment such as a typewriter or word processor, dictating machine, transcriber, or the hire of these, and all associated tapes, disks, ribbons, repairs and maintenance add significantly to writing costs. (*In full or pro rata if bought; in full if hired.*)

Conference attendance

Attendance at conferences, study days, workshops and so on, if directly associated with writing activities, must be costed and records kept. (*In full or pro rata.*)

Photocopying

This includes photocopying parts of books and journals within prescribed limits, purchasing photocopied publications from libraries, and photocopying the final draft of a manuscript. (*In full.*)

Inter-library loan

Inter-library loan costs can be substantial, particularly if a number of books and journals are borrowed through this system whilst researching the subject. (*In full.*)

Thus, the size and range of writing costs are not inconsiderable. The importance of good record keeping is twofold: first, as part of good personal housekeeping and budgeting; secondly, to supply the income tax inspector with evidence of expenditure in order to minimize taxation of royalties. Such evidence will hopefully be accepted and result in a successfully negotiated settlement.

INCOME FROM WRITING

As with writing costs, income derived from writing must be carefully recorded for personal budgeting and income tax purposes. Even small amounts build up and no matter how small are of interest to, and must be declared to, the income tax authorities. The amount of income may range from nil, the amount paid for some journal articles and book reviews, to a modest income from book royalties. In some instances, publishing consultancies for example, the size of the payment received may be negotiable. These examples represent a selection of the types of income paid to writers in the health care professions.

Book reviewing

Payment for writing a book review differs considerably between journals, varying from no payment to a *very* modest one. Virtually all journals allow the reviewer to retain the reviewed book; this is a form of payment which may be regarded as taxable income.

The time involved in reading and writing a review of a book is never fully paid for by financial or 'in kind' income. The real reward is in reading the book, learning from it, and being able to influence the direction of the profession by including appropriate comment.

Articles

A few journals, especially the more prestigious low-circulation ones, do *not* pay a fee to their authors. Indeed, a very small number of journals *charge* authors a fee for publishing in them. Some journals, particularly those that do not pay a fee, may give authors a number of free reprints of the article and a copy of the journal issue in which the article appeared.

Some journals do pay a fairly modest fee which may or may not be related to the length of the article. A typical payment for an average article might be £40–£60, but a small number of high circulation journals pay considerably more. Journals that do not pay a fee make this known. Those that do may not specify the amount until the paper has been submitted and accepted; the author is then offered a payment, to be made on publication.

In general, the payment to writers in professional journals is minimal and rarely enough to cover the costs. Indeed, the choice of where to submit a paper is more often influenced by the reputation of the journal than by possible financial gain.

Books

Payment for writing, or editing, a book usually takes the form of *royalties*, these being an agreed percentage of the publisher's net or gross income from sales of the book. The manner in which royalties are calculated also varies depending on whether the book has an author (or authors) or an editor.

Details of how royalties are to be calculated and paid, the former being a subject for negotiation, are agreed with the publisher as part of the contract. Two typical examples which illustrate the calculation of royalties are: first, to a sole author, and, secondly, to a sole editor.

Author

An author may be paid a percentage of the price received by the publisher. For example, although a book sells to the public for £10, the price paid by the bookseller to the publisher (wholesale price) might be £6. The author might typically expect to receive a 10% royalty on each book sold (60 pence). As a result of the increasing level of discount requested by booksellers, publishers are now less likely to pay an author a percentage of the retail price of the book, that is, a percentage of the published price. Less frequently the author may be paid royalties on the retail price. For example, if the book sells at £10 and the author is paid a 10% royalty, he or she would receive £1 from each book sold.

The amount of royalty paid, as a percentage of either retail or wholesale price varies between publishers and may be increased once a predetermined number of books has been sold. For example a 10% royalty might be paid for the first 3000 copies sold, 12% for the next 3000 and 15% thereafter. If the publisher does not make such an offer, the writer should ask for it.

There are other financial aspects which may be included in the contract such as variations in the payment of royalties on books sold overseas. The frequency and date(s) on which royalties are paid will be specified, normally once or twice a year. A number of free copies of the book, ranging from 5 to 25, may be given to the author in addition to the opportunity to buy additional copies at a reduced cost. As with virtually all aspects of the contract, this item is negotiable prior to signing.

If the book has more than one author, the publisher will distribute royalties equally between them unless the authors agree and formally indicate otherwise.

Editor

If one person is editing a book to which he or she and a number of other writers are contributing, an arrangement similar to the one for authors may apply. However, the distribution of royalties between the editor and contributors requires the following type of additional arrangement.

If the royalty is 10% of the published (retail) price, one-third of that royalty amount may be paid to the editor, the remainder being distributed between all contributors, including the editor, on a pro rata basis. If there are 20 chapters, the writer of each chapter will receive one-twentieth of two-thirds of the 10% royalty. Example 45 shows how such royalties would be calculated for the writer of one chapter if the book had a retail cost of £9.

Example 45

Chapter contributor's royalty payment calculation

$$\frac{£9 \times 10\% \times 66.6\%}{20} = 3 \text{ pence per book sold}$$

An alternative arrangement for paying contributors is to agree on a set fee or single payment which may be calculated on an agreed amount per thousand words, for example. Such a payment may be paid by the editor, or by the publisher and then deducted from royalties paid to the editor. Some contributors may wish to receive a set fee payment; others might prefer royalties. In either case it is the editor who determines the method and amount of payment to contributors in negotiation with them.

Advance payments

The cost of preparing a book manuscript can be considerable, running into several hundred pounds. Because this cost may be beyond the means of some prospective authors and editors, publishers *may* be willing to make a usually small advance against royalties at some point in the manuscript's preparation prior to its publication. However, a publisher might be reluctant to give an advance payment. This attitude is understandable if it is borne in mind that a large number of book proposals are started but never completed. Such advances, if paid, are deducted from the first one, or two, royalty payments. If the proposal is abandoned, the advance must be returned to the publisher.

If a book proposal to which a publisher is attracted has been written but cannot proceed because of lack of finances, the writer should not hesitate to present the publisher with a reasonable and well argued request for an advance.

Consultancy work

In addition to the health care professional employed on a full-time basis, some book and journal publishers employ additional suitably experienced professionals on an ad hoc or retainer basis.

Ad hoc consultancy

Although publishers have a vested interest in maintaining good relationships with their publishing consultants and in paying them a reasonable fee, there is considerable variation in the level of fee paid for pieces of work of similar volume and complexity.

Although *every* piece of consultancy work is unique in content, the following proposition is offered as a guide for publishers and their ad hoc consultants. A possible starting point for negotiation is an hourly payment of one and a half times the present gross hourly earnings of the consultant, or what might be earned if he or she is not working at present. Thus, if the person has a gross annual salary of £20 000, the hourly rate charged to a publisher would be as shown in Example 46.

Example 46 ───

Calculation of hourly charge for consultancy work

$$\frac{£20\,000 \text{ (annual salary)} \times 1.5}{52 \text{ weeks} \times 37 \text{ hours (length of working week)}} = £15.59\text{p per hour}$$

A charge of 150% of the consultant's hourly income for good quality advice, comment and opinion, bearing in mind that the fee will have to cover telephone, postage and typing costs, is both reasonable and appropriate. Clearly, if an individual wishes to negotiate a higher fee, that is quite appropriate provided that the matter is discussed with the publisher in advance of an agreement being made. The writer who is asked to do a job and is offered a fixed payment should inform the publisher of the amount of time the sum will buy, and should make it clear that only that amount of time will be spent on the work. If either party suggests that more time is required, the payment must be adjusted to take account of this.

By using the type of arrangement proposed here, both consultant and publisher will become much more aware of the time and effort needed to do a particular job. It will also go some way towards preventing the type of situation arising in which a colleague of the present author spent hundreds of hours doing a consultancy job for which she was paid approximately 5% of her hourly rate from normal employment.

It is not being suggested that publishers presently underpay their consultants, or that they should be charged unreasonable fees. However, both parties will benefit from a realistic payment system which takes full account of what needs to be done *and* the amount of time needed to do the job.

Consultancy retainer

A second type of remuneration for consultancy work is the payment of an agreed annual retention fee for a specified amount of work. If the volume of work given to the consultant goes beyond a predetermined level, that is, the amount of hours the retainer will buy, additional negotiable ad hoc payments are made.

Public Lending Right

Under the Public Lending Right, payment to authors whose books are lent out by public libraries is made from public funds. Information about this payment, which is only made if authors and books are registered, is available to United Kingdom residents from: Public Lending Right Office, Rayheath House, Prince Regent Street, Stockton on Tees, Cleveland TS18 1DF, England.

INCOME TAX

Part of the reason why meticulous record keeping is so necessary in relation to expenditure and income relating to writing for publication is that it is vital to ensure that appropriate income tax payments (neither too much nor too little) are made. Although the remainder of this chapter deals with a number of aspects of that subject, individual readers will have to ensure personally that they are aware of all the rules and regulations relating to their specific circumstances.

Publishers are usually helpful in response to requests for tax guidance from their authors: indeed some provide a guide for authors that covers taxation on royalties. In addition authors should also feel free to seek advice from the Inland Revenue or from a tax consultant. Needless to say, each contributor to a multiauthored or multiedited work must take individual responsibility for all personal taxation matters.

Articles

Profits from writing articles, that is, the extent to which income exceeds expenditure, or from other 'isolated literary activities' may be stated in a tax return by simply indicating total income and expenditure. For example, if £50 is received for a published article, the profits may be calculated as shown in Example 47.

Example 47

Calculation of profits from published article

Income	Item	Expenditure
£50	Typing	£22.60
	Postage	£1.80
	Telephone	£3.75
	Stationery	£2.55
	Inter-library loan	£6.15
	Total	£36.85
		Profit = £13.15

Thus, the information in Example 47, which must all be supplied to the Inland Revenue, indicates a profit of £13.15 on which income tax will have to be paid. In those cases where expenditure exceeds income, there will be no profit and therefore no tax to pay. If these details cannot be entered on the usual form, they must be included in a covering letter a copy of which must be kept.

Books

Whereas income from articles tends to be a one-off item and the expenditure is confined to the narrow time period in which the paper was written, income and expenditure from a book will be spread over a number of years. In the earlier years there will be expenditure but no income, and in later years income but no expenditure. It is therefore important that the Inland Revenue be informed of expenditure in the first tax return made after the signing of a contract with the publisher. In subsequent years, in addition to an annual statement of expenditure and income, a running total of both items must be submitted. When the running total of income exceeds expenditure, income tax will be due on the balance, that is, on the 'profit'.

Example 48 shows how the above information, in the form of a letter, might be presented. The example, the second annual letter submitted, relates to an imaginary book which has not yet been published, but for which an advance payment was received in 1992.

Example 48

Format of information submitted for income tax purposes

For financial year: 1992–1993

Re: *Health Care in the 21st Century*
   Anticipated publication date: December 1994
   Publisher: Professional Publications, New Town

Personal expenditure associated with above writing activity, 1992–1993

	£
Professional books (pro rata)	amount
Travel associated with writing	amount
Conference costs (pro rata)	amount
Professional journals	amount
Telephone	amount
Stationery, disks, tapes, ribbons, etc.	amount
Home writing costs (% of heating, lighting, mortgage)	amount
Photocopying	amount
Article reprints, inter-library loans	amount
Postage	amount
Typing and secretarial	amount
Indexing	amount
Total expenditure in above period (1992–1993)	£ amount

Income from above writing activity, 1992–1993

Advance payment from professional publications	£ amount

As in previous years, I enclose a running total of expenditure, which started in 1991, and of income, which started in 1992.

Expenditure:	1991–1993	£ amount
Income:	1991–1993	£ amount

If income exceeds expenditure, the balance will be taxed; if expenditure exceeds income, no tax payment should be necessary. Because of the legal implications of providing information for taxation purposes, writers are *urged* to seek specialist advice if in doubt about *any* aspects of the subject. The need to keep accurate and detailed records is self-evident.

A healthy interest in the economics of writing, and in ensuring that a reasonable reward is obtained for quality work, is not only professional but also goes some way towards encouraging a professionally essential activity.

Chapter 23
Teaching and Learning Writing Skills

There are many ways of learning how to write for a professional readership. Some health care professionals undoubtedly have a natural writing talent which enables them to write effortlessly and without being taught. However, the vast majority of health care professionals who write books, contribute to the professional journals, review books and so on, are self-taught, having learned by trial and error and with considerable effort.

As with many subjects there are individuals who, for a variety of reasons, prefer to learn and develop writing skills privately and without the perceived constraints and disadvantages of 'being taught', or participating in collecting learning. They may find this book, including this chapter, of value in their endeavours.

Many others, perhaps even the majority, would probably prefer involvement in a teaching/learning activity which will accelerate and improve the quality of the learning process. One way of developing writing skills is to participate in a structured programme, in the form of a workshop for example. This chapter provides a structure for such a workshop or series of workshops.

Different individuals will have varying needs depending on their previous career development, the career stage reached, and future writing aspirations. For example, qualified staff who have successfully passed all exams and coursework may have little need of a workshop on that topic, although teaching staff may profit from it. However, student entrants into the professions would probably benefit from being taught this subject in a workshop or some other appropriate format. The same selective principle applies to virtually all topics covered in this book; if the individual has successfully published a book, journal article or book reviews, that person is probably better qualified to be a teacher than a workshop participant.

If a series of workshops is offered, perhaps in a geographical area or place of work, it would be prudent to allow participants to select and attend those in which they wished to participate and to avoid those subjects in which they are proficient.

Decisions about the amount of time required to teach and learn each of the topics is a matter for individual teachers and students groups. However, this book provides a suggested time allocation that is based on the author's experience of each subject in workshops. The optimum size of a workshop group is between six and ten; less than six is economically expensive and inhibits the volume of discussion material; more than ten reduces too far the amount of individualized attention available to participants. The upper limit of ten participants is central to the necessary reliance on demonstrations and practical work.

The suggested learning objectives and exercises are for demonstration only and can be replaced by any of a number of other appropriate forms of practical work.

The following suggested workshop structure is based on the content of this book, which is not, and cannot be, designed to meet all the needs of all health care professionals. Where subject gaps are identified, they can be accommodated in an extended structure. Each topic is followed by examples of the teaching/learning methods that may be used.

Writing and professionalism: Prior reading/discussion/practical.
Time: Three hours, including practical work.
Participants: All health care professionals who do not yet have a well developed record in writing for publication.
Workshop leader: A member of the profession from which participants are drawn, or from any of the disciplines if the workshop is multidisciplinary. The leader will have considerable professional *and* writing experience, including a track record in professional publications.
Learning objectives: Participants will be able to contribute fully to a discussion of 'writing and professionalism' and write a two-page paper entitled 'Writing for publication, a professional necessity?'.

Writing opportunities: Prior reading/discussion.
Time: Three hours, including practical work.
Participants: All health care professionals who do not yet have a well developed record in writing for publication.
Workshop leaders: As for 'Writing and professionalism', together with staff member from publishing house (books or journals).
Learning objectives: Participants will be able to contribute fully to a discussion of writing opportunities and to prepare a summary of personal writing activities planned for the next five years.

Resources for writing: Prior reading/discussion.
Time: three hours, including practical work.
Participants: Those who intend to develop writing skills, including for professional publication.
Workshop leader: As for 'Writing and professionalism'.
Learning objectives: Participants will be able to contribute fully to a discussion of resources for writing, and to list and briefly describe these in a short paper. Students will also be able to detail the range of resources available to them locally, including in their place of work.

Writing style and structure: Prior reading/discussion/demonstration/ practical.
Time: Four hours, including practical work.
Participants: Those who intend to develop writing skills, including for professional publishing.
Workshop leader: As for 'Writing and professionalism'.
Learning objectives: Participants will be able to write a 1000-word piece of work incorporating a range of appropriate aspects of style and structure. They will also be able to write a two-page critique of the style and structure of an article from a health care journal. The critique will demonstrate the strengths and weaknesses in the article's structure and writing style, and include suggestions for rectifying the latter.

References: Prior reading/discussion/demonstration/practical.
Time: Four hours, including practical work.
Participants: All health care professionals who are not proficient in the use of the Harvard and numerical reference systems.
Workshop leader: As for 'Writing and professionalism'.
Learning objectives: Participants will be able to write a short paper incorporating six references (three books and three articles) using the Harvard system. The essay will be followed by a formal reference list and a brief annotated bibliography. Participants will be able to write a second short essay and reference list using the numerical system.

Literature search: Prior reading/discussion/demonstration/practical.
Time: Six hours (full day), including practical work.
Participants All health care professionals who are not proficient in carrying out a literature search, and in the use of the Harvard and numerical reference systems.
Workshop leaders: (a) as for 'Writing and professionalism' *or* an experienced researcher from a relevant profession; *and* (b) a librarian specializing in relevant health care literature.
Note: Participants will need access to the manual and/or bibliographic tools discussed in Chapter 6, 'Literature search'.
Learning objectives: Participants will be able to undertake a literature search of a selected relevant topic, using three or more of the searching tools described in Chapter 6 (Literature search), and compile a bibliography of ten or more references.

Literature review: Prior reading/discussion/demonstration/practical.
Time: Four hours, including practical work.
Participants: All health care professionals who are not proficient at writing a literature review.
Workshop leader: (a) as for 'Writing and professionalism', *or* (b) an experienced researcher from a relevant profession.

Note: Participants will need access to a comprehensive selection of literature in their professional subject area.
Learning objectives: Participants will be able to write a 500-word critical review and evaluation of at least five pieces of literature identified in the literature search.

Illustrations: Prior reading/discussion/demonstration/practical.
Time: Three hours, including practical work.
Participants: All health care professionals who are not proficient in the construction of illustrations.
Workshop leader: As for 'Writing and professionalism'.
Learning objectives: Participants will be able to demonstrate how five pieces of allocated information in prose form can be well presented in illustrative form *or* write a short essay showing how five illustrative techniques are used appropriately.

Coursework and examinations: Prior reading/discussion/demonstration/practical.
Time: Two hours, including practical work.
Participants: Students and teaching staff.
Workshop leader: Lecturer or examiner.
Learning objectives: Participants will demonstrate, by writing detailed examination answer and coursework structures, that they are familiar with the general principles discussed in Chapter 9. Each section of the structure will include an indication of general content and of length.

Books: Prior reading/discussion/demonstration/practical.
Time: Four hours, including practical work.
Participants: Senior health care professionals who are considering becoming the author or editor of a book.
Workshop leader: A member of any of the professions from which participants are drawn who has considerable experience as an author or editor of professional textbooks.
Learning objectives: Participants will be able to construct a first draft of a book proposal, including answers to the 'Questionnaire Sent to Prospective Authors' presented in Chapter 10. They will also be able to write a two-page critique of the structural and organizational strengths and weaknesses of a textbook with which they are familiar in their discipline, and suggest how the weaknesses can be rectified.

Publishing consultancies: Prior reading/discussion/practical.
Time: Three hours, including practical work.
Participants: Senior health care professionals with publishing experience who are considering publishing consultancy work.
Workshop leader: A member of any health care discipline who has experience in publishing consultancy work.

Learning objectives: Participants will be able to prepare a letter to a book publisher making a case for being considered for consultancy work. They will also be able to select a journal article and, whilst assuming it has been sent to them in manuscript form by a publisher for review, answer the questions which have been set out in Chapter 11.

Checking, proofreading and indexing: Prior reading/discussion/ practical.
Time: Three hours, including practical work.
Participants: Health care professionals who are considering writing either articles or books.
Workshop leader: A member of any health care profession with experience in writing articles and/or books for publication.
Learning objectives: Participants will be able to select an article from a professional journal and write an index to include all relevant indexable items. They will also be able to proofread a two-page paper containing a number of deliberate errors, and indicate the necessary changes using the proof correction marks in Example 32.

Research reports: Prior reading/discussion/practical.
Time: Three hours, including practical work.
Participants: Health care professionals who anticipate undertaking a piece of research, or who have embarked on a study but have not written the report.
Workshop leader: A member of any health care profession who has written a number of research reports.
Learning objectives: Participants will be able to write a possible structure, with an outline of content, of their research or intended research.

Dissertations and theses: Prior reading/discussion/practical.
Time: Four hours, including practical work.
Participants: Health care professionals who are, or who are anticipating, undertaking a piece of research as part of an academic course or higher degree requirement.
Workshop leader: A member of any health care profession who has successfully completed a higher degree and has supervised one or more of these.
Learning objectives: Participants will be able to select a completed dissertation or thesis with which they are familiar and critically evaluate it in terms of style, presentation and structure; and write a possible structure for an actual or intended dissertation or thesis.

Articles: Prior reading/discussion/practical.
Time: Four hours, including practical work.
Participants: All health care professionals.

Workshop leader: A member of any health care profession with extensive experience of writing articles for publication.

Learning objectives: Participants will be able to identify a topic to form the basis of a manuscript for submission to an editor, write the first draft structure of the article and, if time allows, add some content.

Curriculum vitae and résumé: Prior reading/discussion/practical.

Time: Four hours, including practical work.

Participants: All health care professionals who have not yet personally written their curriculum vitae.

Workshop leader: A member of any health care profession who has a well developed, personally written and regularly updated curriculum vitae.

Learning objectives: Participants will be able to write a detailed structure, with first draft content, of their curriculum vitae.

Book reviews: Prior reading/discussion/practical.

Time: Four hours, including practical work.

Participants: All health care professionals who intend to become book reviewers.

Workshop leader: Any health care professional with considerable book reviewing experience.

Learning objectives: Participants will be able to write a convincing letter to a journal editor requesting that they be considered as a book reviewer; and write a 300-word first draft of a review of a professional book with which they are familiar.

Writing and presenting a speech: Prior reading/discussion/practical.

Time: Four hours, including practical work.

Participants: All health care professionals, other than those with wide experience of the subject.

Workshop leader: Any health care professional with wide experience of public speaking to professional audiences.

Learning objectives: Participants will be able to write a well structured 10-minute talk on a professional subject of their choice; and, if requested, present the prepared speech for critical evaluation.

Writing a research proposal: Prior reading/discussion/practical.

Time: Four hours, including practical work.

Participants: All health care professionals who intend or are likely to undertake a research project.

Workshop leader: Any health care professional with considerable experience as a researcher and research supervisor.

Learning objectives: Participants will be able to construct a two- to three-page first draft proposal on a subject of their choice.

Travel scholarship application: Prior reading/discussion/practical.
Time: Three hours, including practical work.
Participants: All health care professionals.
Workshop leader: Any health care professional who has successfully submitted two or more travel scholarship applications.
Learning objectives: Participants will be able to write a first draft of a research scholarship application.

Writing technology: Prior reading/discussion/practical.
Time: Seven hours (full day), including practical work.
Participants: All health care professionals who are not proficient in using a word processor.
Workshop leader: Anyone with word processing skills and with teaching experience in the subject.
Note: All participants will need sole access to a word processor for the duration of this workshop session.
Learning objectives: Participants will become sufficiently proficient to independently write a one-page item on a word processor. (Grammatical and typographical errors may be disregarded.)

Economics of writing: Prior reading/discussion/practical.
Time: Two hours, including practical work.
Participants: All health care professionals who are, or anticipate, receiving royalties from writing, editing or contributing to a textbook, or from any other professional writing activity.
Workshop leader: Any health care professional who has incurred expenditure, and derived income from, writing for professional publication, and/or who is familiar with basic income tax implications.
Learning objectives: Participants will be able to document the expenditure and income derived from a prescribed range of writing activities.

There can be no blueprint for teaching and learning any subject, and writing for health care professions is no exception to this rule. This chapter contains only examples of how the material in the preceding 22 chapters might be structured as part of an educational package. Some professionals do not need this type of assistance; they write well and will continue to do so. However, the teaching assistance of the successful minority will undoubtedly help the very large majority who have the desire and potential to develop their writing skills generally and to contribute to the professional literature in particular.

Epilogue

The factors that encourage professionals to go on writing beyond the point at which their educational system makes it compulsory are many and varied. This is particularly true of the factors that motivate writing for publication, a challenging and yet rewarding activity.

Professionals involved with health care are motivated to write and publish by a mixture of altruism and egocentricity. There can be no doubt that seeing one's name in print for the first time, in the form of authorship of a publication, is an extremely rewarding experience. However, the ego becomes decreasingly stimulated as more and more publishing success inevitably follows.

In the longer term the drive to publish changes in its emphasis. Whereas, initially, ego satisfaction is *probably* more evident than altruism, the balance reverses as experience in publishing increases. Experienced authors are often genuinely influenced by a desire to help their professional colleagues deliver a better quality of service to their patients/clients. Arguably, this desire to serve is an essential ingredient of professionalism.

A modest amount of financial reward *may* be achieved by writing professional articles and books, particularly if full attention is paid to the economics of writing. Indeed, it is important that a realistic (even commercial) approach be taken to financial issues. In this way contributors to the literature will be better able to afford to continue their very necessary work.

Throughout this book, the right and responsibility of all professionals to contribute to their literature has been emphasized. It has been proposed that all professionals, with appropriate assistance in relation to the mechanics of writing, have an important role to play. This assistance can take the form of a self-teaching programme, possibly with assistance from teachers or colleagues, or of a more formally structured educational experience such as may be offered during a writing workshop.

My experience with the writing/workshop approach has been positive and fruitful, considerable advances in writing skill being achieved even in a short period. This type of programme is of particular relevance to professionals who have been 'out of school' for some time and who wish to start writing for publication. To those who decide to learn for themselves I wish 'Bon Voyage'. For those who decide to offer or attend a writing workshop, I hope that this book is a useful starting point.

Just as a journey begins with the first step, a manuscript begins with the first word.

Recommended Reference Texts

Allen, R.E. (Editor) (1990) *The Oxford Writer's Dictionary.* Oxford, Oxford University Press.

Black, A. & C. (1993) *The Writers' and Artists' Yearbook.* London, A. & C. Black.

Blackwell Scientific Publications (1989) *Guidelines for Authors.* Oxford, Blackwell Scientific Publications.

Bryson, B. (1991) *The Penguin Dictionary for Writers and Editors.* London, Penguin.

Butler, P. (Editor) (1991) *The Economist Style Guide.* London, Business Books.

Clark, C. (1990) *Photocopying from Books and Journals.* London, The British Copyright Council.

Day, R.A. (1989) *How to Write and Publish a Scientific Paper* (3rd ed). Cambridge, Cambridge University Press.

De Freitas, D. (1990) *The British Council's Guide to the Law of Copyright and Rights in Performances.* London, The British Copyright Council.

Hart, H. (1992) *Hart's Rules* (39th ed). Oxford, Oxford University Press.

Isaacs, A., Daineth, J. & Martin, E. (Editors) (1992) *Dictionary for Scientific Writers and Editors.* Oxford, Oxford University Press.

Jenkins, S. (Editor) (1992) *The Times Guide to English Style and Usage.* London, Times Books.

Kahn, J. (1991) *How to Write and Speak Better.* London, Reader's Digest Books.

O'Connor, M. (1991) *Writing Successfully in Science.* London, HarperCollins.

The Publishers Association (1991) *Directory of Publishing. United Kingdom, Commonwealth and Overseas.* London, Cassell.

Quilliam, S. & Grove-Stephenson, I. (1990) *Into Print.* London, BBC Books.

Rimmer, S. (1991) *The Home Office Computer Book.* San Francisco, Sybex.

The Society of Authors (1991) *Quick Guide: Publishing Contracts.* London, The Society of Authors. Also by the same author/publisher, *Quick Guides* on: *Authors' Agents*; *Copyright and Moral Rights*; *The Protection of Titles*; *Copyrights after Your Death*; *Libel*; *Income Tax*; *Buying a Word-Processor*; *Permissions*; *Artistic Work and Photographs*; *Guidelines for Authors of Medical Books*.

Turner, B. (Editor) (1992) *The Writer's Handbook.* London, Macmillan.

Urdang, L. (1991) *The Oxford Thesaurus. An A–Z Dictionary of Synonyms.* Oxford, Clarendon Press.

Index

Page numbers in **bold** indicate whole chapters.

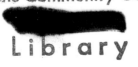